THE
KETO
CURE

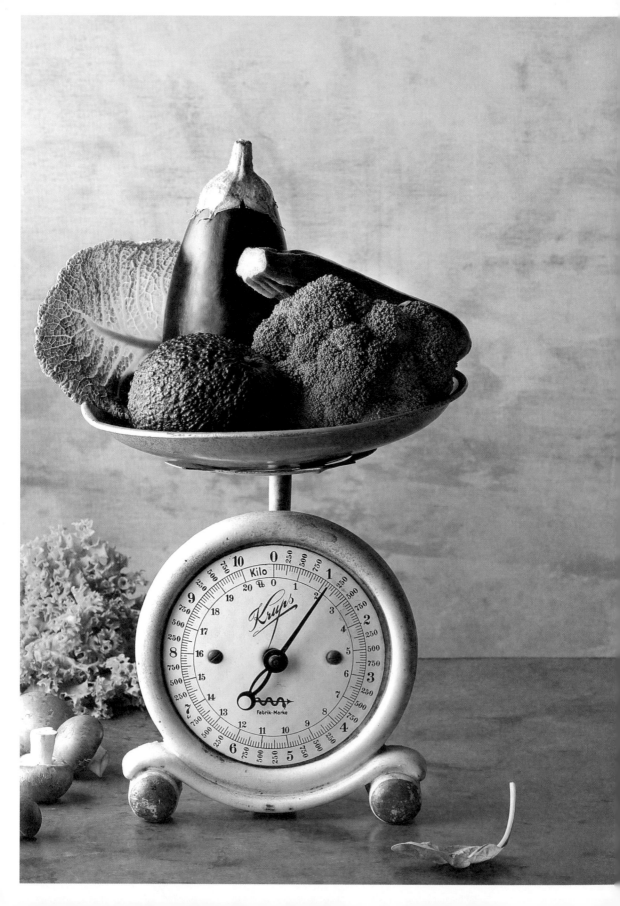

Professor Jürgen Vormann
with Nico Stanitzok

THE KETO CURE

The Essential 28-Day Low-Carb
High-Fat Weight-Loss Plan

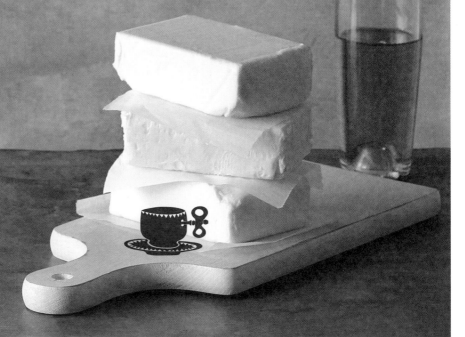

CONTENTS

The (v) beside the recipe identifies a vegetarian dish

FOREWORD

I first studied nutritional science over 30 years ago and have been researching and teaching it ever since. In hardly any other field of science has our understanding of what is healthy for us changed as fundamentally as in relation to nutrition.

For a long time, a low-fat diet was considered synonymous with being healthy. People cut back on fat and made up for lost calories by eating (supposedly healthier) carbohydrates. Then, research started to show that a high-carb diet has the potential to lead to serious health complications, such as obesity and type 2 diabetes, two of the most prevalent health problems in modern society. As a result, the low-carbohydrate diet became a highly popular alternative.

But eating fat to stay slim? Well, yes. Today we know that a high-fat diet can actually be beneficial, particularly if you are overweight. While it understandably feels counterintuitive to eat more fat, the latest scientific evidence shows that a low-carbohydrate high-fat diet combined with exercise will help regulate your metabolism and give you back control over your weight.

Because eating habits are shaped and consolidated over long periods of time, it can be difficult for us to make the fundamental shift from a carbohydrate-based to a high-fat diet—not least because of a lack of kitchen inspiration. This is where we come in. In *The Keto Cure* we will help you adapt to the Low-Carb High-Fat diet (LCHF for short), with plenty of delicious recipes to show you the way. My friend and colleague Nico Stanitzok has based his career on his passion for tasty, nutritionally-balanced food. For this book he has developed recipes suitable for everyday life which are low in carbs, high in fat, and will keep you satisfied and healthy.

This book, and our 28-day program, is a starting point. People who want to lose weight will see the results quickly but the main benefit for everyone is that this is a medium- to long-term healthy diet-option, in contrast to the low-carb, high-protein diet which has several negative impacts on general health. In the pages that follow, you will discover why the LCHF approach is the key to successful weight loss.

Dr. Jürgen Vormann

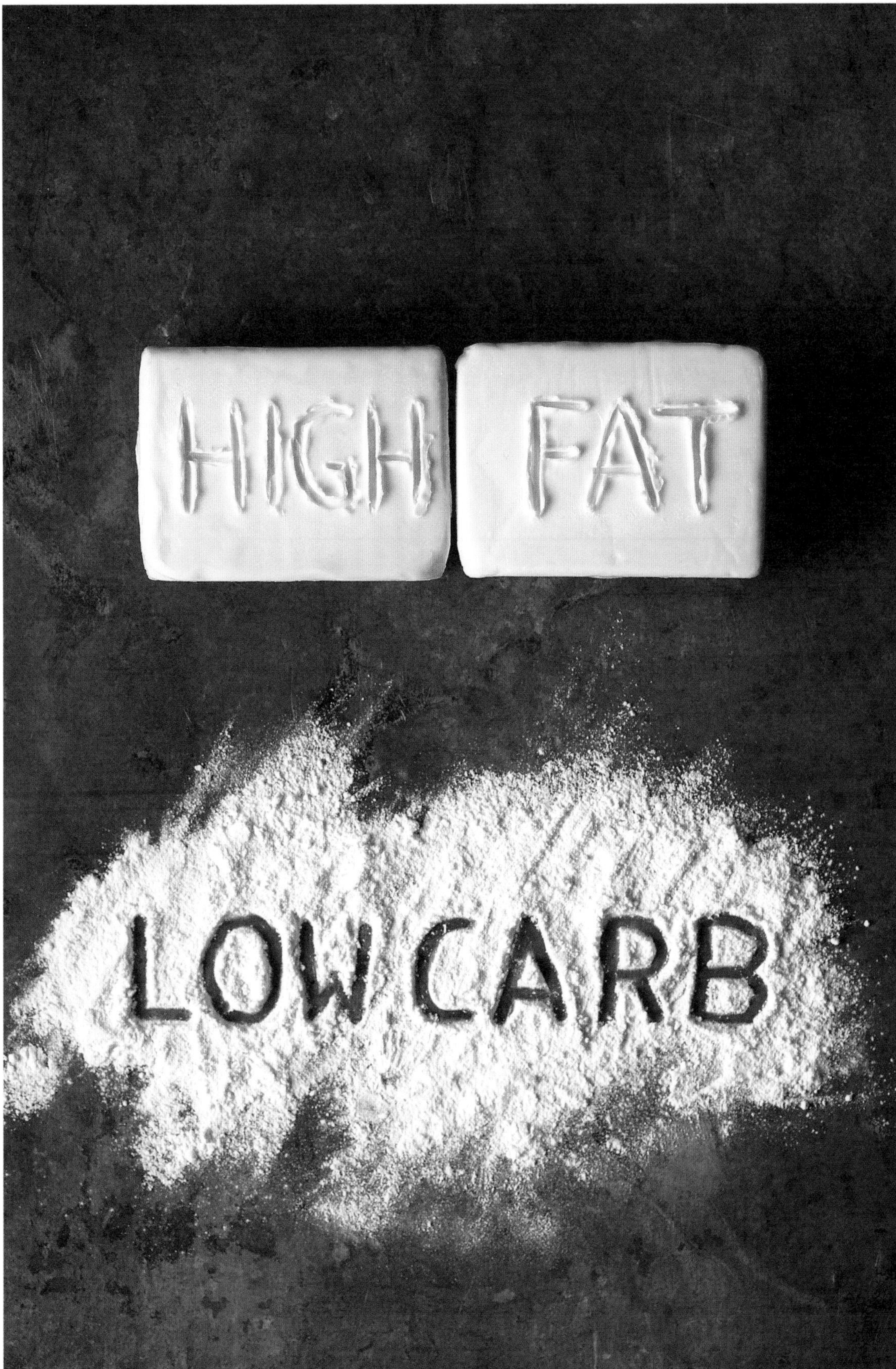
HIGH FAT
LOW CARB

WHY LOW CARB HIGH FAT?

In order for our bodies to function properly, our diet has to include a regular supply of energy from one of three sources: carbohydrate, fat and protein. If we restrict one of the nutrients in this mix, but want to maintain the same energy intake, we have to make up the shortfall by consuming more of one of the other energy sources.

Some low-carb diets rely on substituting protein for the missing carbohydrate calories – so you might eat some extra steak in place of pasta or bread. The abundance of meat has made this diet attractive to many people, especially men, at least for a time. But there are certain pitfalls that can limit the benefits of these kinds of diets; when the amino acids that make up the proteins are broken down, the body produces intermediate products that form carbohydrates. The end result of this is that consuming too much protein indirectly increases your supply of carbohydrates. High protein consumption can also put a strain on the body's acid-base balance.

MORE FAT, LESS PROTEIN

If we don't substitute the calories missing from carbohydrates with protein, the only other option is fat. In a low-carb diet, your body burns more of its own fat stores, which is exactly the effect you want if you are trying to lose weight. Reducing your carbohydrate intake means your muscle cells in particular burn more fat to generate energy. The heart, for instance, can derive almost all its energy requirements from fatty acids.

A low-carb high-fat (LCHF) diet has an additional advantage over the low-carb high-protein diet: by increasing the intake of fat at the same time as limiting carbohydrates, it pushes the body to produce ketones. In a traditional diet, these chemicals are only present in the body in tiny quantities. But they are an effective substitute for carbohydrates, and all cells can use ketones as a rapid form of fuel.

Since we usually have substantial fat stores in our bodies, it is always possible for our body to produce ketones. However, ketones are only created when the body's metabolism switches to fat burning, particularly in the liver. As soon as we start consuming significant quantities of carbohydrates, our metabolism switches back to using glucose; once this occurs, we start building up fat stores again and ketosis ceases. Reducing your carbohydrate consumption in the short term will not produce a long-term effect, so the crucial thing for maintaining your target weight is to reduce carbohydrates on a sustained basis.

Decades of warnings against excessive fat consumption have certainly made their mark. Many of us who want to lose weight find it counterintuitive to increase our fat intake. But this diet has already helped a great many people; it will help you, too.

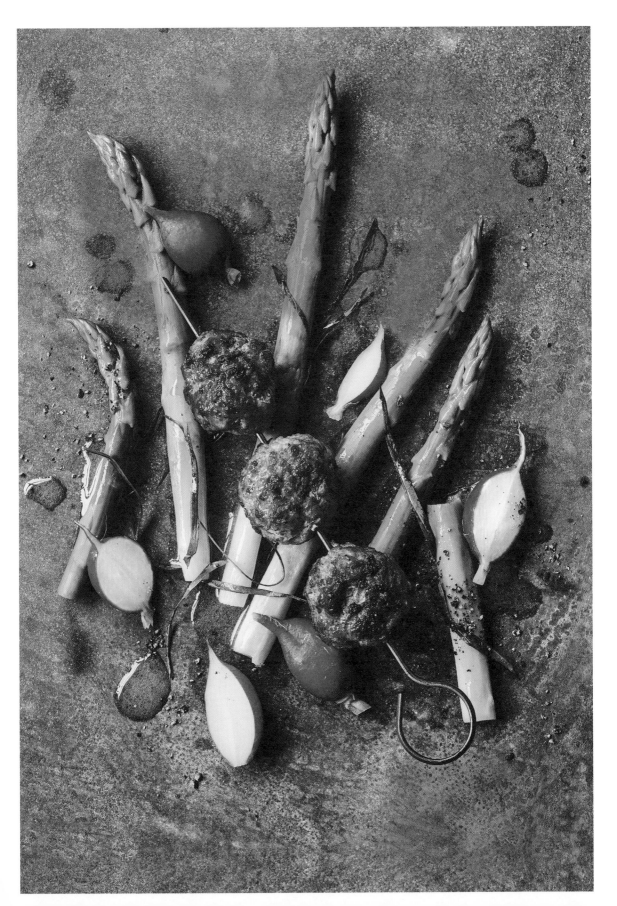

FATTENING CARBOHYDRATES

Carbohydrates are absolutely essential for our metabolism. But in excess quantities they overwhelm our blood sugar levels and encourage our bodies to store fat. In order to lose weight, we have to address carbohydrate consumption.

Our metabolism releases insulin to control blood sugar concentrations, ensuring there is always enough glucose in our bloodstream while also preventing excess. Any excess sugar in the blood is rapidly removed – our muscles then burn (and store some of) this glucose. But if we continue to supply the body with glucose, for example, in the case of a carbohydrate-rich meal, then we hit the scenario we want to avoid: the excess sugar is no longer stored as carbohydrates and is instead converted into fat.

Often the food we eat does not consist purely of carbohydrates; it also contains fat. In this case, our metabolism has enough glucose available that it does not need to use the fat we are eating as a source of energy – so off it goes, straight into our fat stores. Only once glucose levels in our bloodstream are back to normal can our body use this fat. However, a decrease in blood sugar will send an unmistakable signal to our body that additional supplies are required: we become hungry. If we then eat more carbohydrates, our body uses these first and the stored fat stays in our fatty tissues. It's a vicious circle that ultimately leads to obesity. Of course, you can break the cycle by refusing to give in to your hunger – but this is far from easy. Or you can stimulate glucose consumption through exercise, but in order to lose weight successfully, physical activity needs to supplement an existing calorie deficit.

INSULIN AS THE CONTROLLER

The hormone insulin plays a central role in controlling glucose metabolism. It enables glucose to be absorbed by the cells in our muscles and liver and ensures that the metabolic processing in our brain functions correctly. Whenever glucose enters our bloodstream following a meal, the pancreas releases insulin to channel that glucose into our cells and inhibit fat burning. After a carbohydrate-rich meal, our body produces a lot of insulin, which continues to act in the bloodstream even after many hours. This means that if we want to program our metabolism to burn fat, it is crucial to keep insulin levels as low as possible. This also helps protect our capacity. If we push our body to produce a lot of insulin over a sustained period, the result can be insulin resistance, where the metabolism barely responds, or fails to respond at all, to insulin. This leads to obesity and diabetes.

LESS IS MORE

Simply put, the fewer carbs you eat, the better! On the LCHF diet, only about 50 grams (1¾ ounces) of carbohydrates per day are needed to meet the brain's requirements. When resting, our brain requires roughly 20 per cent of the calories we consume – for 2000 calories per day, that amounts to about 400 calories. This corresponds to approximately 100 grams (3½ ounces) of carbohydrates. As we reprogram our metabolic system, the absolute glucose requirement (the minimum amount needed for brain function) falls to roughly 50 grams (1¾ ounces) because around half of the brain's energy needs can be met indirectly by breaking down fat. Individuals vary in terms of their metabolism and energy requirements, but over time you will find out what your minimum requirements are.

NOT ALL CARBS ARE BAD

It's not just a question of how many carbohydrates foods contain, but also how quickly each particular carbohydrate is converted into glucose in the bloodstream. This is called a food's glycaemic index, which describes how quickly the carbohydrates in any food are broken down in the intestine and channelled into the blood.

The guidelines are relatively simple: cereal products, potatoes, rice and sugar are prohibited or only to be consumed in very small quantities. Carbohydrates should really come almost exclusively from vegetables, salad and a bit of fruit – these are the 'good' carb sources (see page 12).

HIDDEN CARBOHYDRATES

Ready-made sauces, yoghurts and juices often contain carbohydrates where you would least expect them. They are also found in sausages, shop-bought meatballs, fish dishes and any products coated in breadcrumbs. Even pulses and sweet fruit contain considerable quantities. If you eat carbohydrates these should ideally come from vegetables and fruit, rather than from grains and potatoes. But you should also be wary of hidden carbs. Oysters for example – unlike other fish – have a relatively high carb count at five per cent. So do garlic and onions. Always check the labelling on processed foods: you may be surprised to see where the carbs are coming from.

Be careful with prepared foods such as egg salad, dressings and sauces: sugar is often added as a flavour enhancer. The more processed the product, the greater the likelihood it will contain hidden carbohydrates in the form of sugar and starch. A salad, often considered a healthy alternative, may actually become a calorie and carbohydrate trap because of its dressing. To be on the safe side, prepare sauces and dressings yourself and check the ingredients when you eat out in restaurants. Ketchup is a whopping 25 per cent carbs. While fruit is an important component of the LCHF diet, bear in mind that not all fruits are equal. Pears, for example, are 12 per cent carb. While bananas – that sports person's favourite – are actually 20 per cent carb.

Nuts make a quick and easy snack for in-between meals and on-the-go. Since nuts are naturally very high in calories, it is important to pay attention to the quantities. Macadamia nuts are ideal for a ketogenic diet, being particularly high in fat while comparatively low in carbohydrate, making them a great source of energy. Brazil nuts and almonds are also good options, but some nuts, such as walnuts, should be consumed in moderation and others, such as cashews, avoided completely.

GOOD CARBOHYDRATES

If you are going to consume carbohydrates, wherever possible these should come from vegetables and fruit. Here you'll find the carbohydrate sources that fit best in a LCHF diet.

① FRUIT

Contain important vitamins and minerals that are essential on a LCHF diet. They also provide us with other healthy substances such as antioxidants. This is particularly the case for strongly coloured varieties of fruit, like berries, papaya or apricots. Simple reminder: the sweeter the fruit, the less suitable it is for LCHF. Older apple or pear varieties, which can be found at farmer's markets for instance, usually contain less sugar than newer varieties that have been cultivated for their high sugar content. Quinces are also relatively low in sugar. The same is true of citrus fruits such as grapefruits and lemons. Make sure you eat fruit that has been processed as little as possible, because all too often sugar is added during processing. Frozen fruit is great, too, as it is harvested when perfectly ripe. Frozen berries are a particularly wonderful daily addition to the menu and have a high nutritional value.

② VEGETABLES

Contain lots of vitamins, minerals and alkaline substances that are particularly important on a LCHF diet. The daily quantity of carbohydrates should be derived predominantly from vegetables. All types of cabbage, green salad, cucumbers, spinach, tomatoes, asparagus, broccoli, aubergines, courgettes, peppers, onions and mushrooms can be eaten freely. Take advantage of the high fat content of avocados and olives. Frozen vegetables are a healthy and practical alternative to fresh produce. Be more restrained when it comes to root vegetables, such as potatoes, sweet potatoes, beetroots and carrots, because plants store carbohydrates in roots and bulbs.

③ PULSES

Are a good source of high-quality protein, but lentils and chickpeas in particular also contain lots of carbohydrates. If pulses are to be on the menu, you should preferably stick to peas and beans, which are lower in carbohydrates than other pulses.

④ ALTERNATIVE FLOURS

Can replace carbohydrate-rich ingredients such as sugar, potatoes, rice and cereals, which are less suitable for the LCHF diet. Almond flour is a great flour substitute that contains just 6 grams (about ¼ ounce) of carbohydrates per 100 grams (2½ ounces). You can use it with sweeteners in baked items, though you will find that your appetite for sweet things gradually diminishes over time. Other nut flours such as ground linseed, pumpkin seeds or pine nuts are also good alternatives to cereal flours.

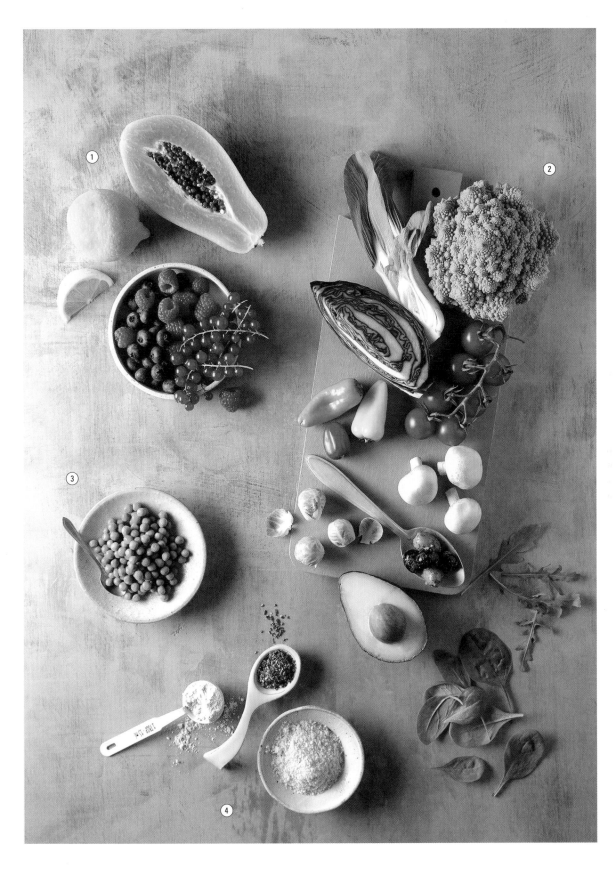

EAT PROTEIN SPARINGLY

It's tempting to make up for the calories saved on carbohydrates in the form of large portions of meat, fish or cheese. But this results in a far higher protein consumption than the roughly 1 gram per kilo (about 2¼ ounces) of body weight required each day. On a low-carb diet, the upper limit should be around 2 grams protein per kilo of body weight. And this can be reached in no time: for someone weighing 75 kilos (165 pounds), this works out at roughly 150 grams (5 ounces) protein. When expressed in calories, this corresponds to roughly 600 per day.

THE DARK SIDE OF PROTEINS

Proteins are composed of individual components known as amino acids. We need amino acids as fuel and as a building material, for example for our muscles. Amino acids contain certain chemical elements, especially nitrogen and sulfur, which have to be excreted via the kidneys because we cannot convert everything into endogenous protein (protein that ensures cells function correctly). This is why excess protein intake puts a strain on our kidneys. A diet based exclusively on protein is actually impossible in the long term, as our kidneys have a limited ability to eliminate nitrogen.

The sulfur contained in protein poses additional problems. Sulfur can only be eliminated from the body in the form of sulfuric acid via the kidneys. Excess quantities of sulfuric acid can contribute significantly to harmful hyperacidity in the body. From around age 30 the excretion capacity of our kidneys becomes more limited, and from this point on there is an unavoidable reduction in kidney capacity of approximately 1 per cent for each year of life.

Due to this continual decline in kidney function, older people can be particularly affected by excess acidity and its negative consequences. The body attempts to compensate for any hyperacidity by releasing more and more alkaline components from the bone structure. Unfortunately, this also results in vital calcium being lost from the bones; the risk of osteoporosis increases and the bones become less stable. An exposure to acidity can also result in painful changes to connective tissue. Ketones are also acidic, which means the aim must be to keep the quantity of additional acid produced to a minimum.

For this reason, a LCHF diet with high quantities of protein is ill-advised. There is another important reason, too: some of the amino acids that make up proteins can be converted into glucose. The proportion of these amino acids is the same across all foods containing protein, so it isn't possible to specifically avoid these proteins. Just like carbohydrates, they can also trigger an insulin response – an effect we want to avoid.

High protein intake is often synonymous with high levels of meat consumption. In addition to animal protein, this means that large quantities of nucleic acids are consumed, and when these are broken down uric acid is produced. This can lead to problems when converting to a LCHF diet, because ketones and uric acid end up competing for the same excretion systems in the kidneys. This can result in obstructions and inhibit excretion. So, at the start of a LCHF diet, the concentration of uric acid in the blood may increase. If a lot of meat is also consumed, the effect is further exacerbated.

Although uric acid is an important antioxidant in the blood and an increase is generally beneficial, this is not the case if you are already suffering from gout, as gout is caused by elevated uric acid levels. If this applies to you, please consult your physician before making any dietary changes. With normal protein intake, kidney function will adapt after four to six weeks and uric acid levels will normalize.

Increased protein intake is possible on a low-carb regime, but not to the extent that would be required to make up for the calorie deficit caused by omitting carbohydrates. Only higher fat consumption can do this.

SLIMMING WITH FAT?

It seems obvious why the original aim for losing weight was to eat less fat. After all, 1 gram of fat contains more than double the calories of either carbohydrates or protein. By reducing fat, you can cut back on significantly more calories than through the same quantity of proteins or carbohydrates. However, we now know that fat is particularly crucial for feeling full. The same quantity of calories in the form of carbohydrates is significantly less filling than those from fat.

Fat has long been blamed for causing various health conditions, especially heart disease. However, we have now established that important research in this area was misinterpreted. For many decades, people have been attempting to lower high cholesterol values (regarded as the main cause of heart attacks) by reducing fat intake. Blood cholesterol levels can be reduced in this way, but this also impacts HDL cholesterol, which we now regard as beneficial to our health. Based on current knowledge, a diet that is high in fat and low in carbohydrates does not constitute a risk in terms of cardiovascular disease. Whether it actually reduces the general risk is a question requiring further research – but initial scientific studies certainly point in this direction.

NOT ALL FATS ARE EQUAL

Needless to say, the kind of fat you eat is hugely important: not all fats are equal. The very fats that have so long been stigmatized are ideally suited for the LCHF diet thanks to their special metabolic state. Long, medium or short-chain? Saturated or unsaturated? These terms crop up repeatedly in association with fats. But what do they mean?

In terms of their chemical make-up, fatty acids are described with reference to the length of their chains, on the one hand, and the nature of their bonds, on the other. Fats with single bonds are described as saturated, while those with double bonds are categorized as unsaturated fats. Chain length and bonding characteristics don't just determine the chemical characteristics of fats, they are also relevant when it comes to nutritional value. One indicator of what kind of fat we are dealing with is its consistency: fats with a higher proportion of unsaturated, long-chain fatty acids are liquid at room temperature, those with saturated fatty acids are solid.

UNSATURATED FATTY ACIDS

Unsaturated fatty acids are important for our metabolism and are known to be beneficial for our health. These include the omega-3 group of fatty acids, but also the monounsaturated oleic acids (of which there are particularly large quantities in olive oil) and the doubly unsaturated linoleic acids (especially prevalent in safflower and grape-seed oil). Omega-3 fatty acids have a particularly beneficial impact on cell membrane structure: these are found in oily sea fish.

Another important source of omega-3 fatty acids is offered by milk, dairy products, meat, sausage, bacon and other products from animals that are allowed to graze on natural pasture. Omega-3 fatty acids from grass are concentrated in these foods, which is why butter from pasture-reared cows also contains a significant proportion of these healthy fats. In addition, olive oil is good for us because of its high levels of monounsaturated oleic acids.

Maintaining a good balance in our diet between plenty of omega-3 fatty acids and minimal omega-6 fatty acids keeps us healthy and protects against illnesses such as cardiovascular disease and arteriosclerosis. Even once conditions like this have developed, and their associated symptoms of inflammation and pain are evident (as with rheumatism, for instance), a high intake of omega-3 with restricted omega-6 fatty acids can have a beneficial impact. Sufficient quantities of omega-3 fatty acids can significantly inhibit the formation of certain pain mediators, known as prostaglandins.

SATURATED FATTY ACIDS

A certain notoriety has been acquired by fats with saturated fatty acids, which are chemically stable and barely change when heated. These fats are claimed to have a negative impact on cholesterol levels, but with LCHF these effects are avoided as the fats are broken down very quickly to produce energy.

As a result, animal products with saturated fats from butter, lard or bacon can be safely included in a LCHF diet. Saturated fats are rare in the plant domain. There are only two varieties with a high proportion of unsaturated fats that are relevant from a nutritional perspective: coconut oil and palm kernel oil (not to be confused with palm oil).

MCT FATS

Medium-chain fatty acids, or MCTs for short, offer a crucial benefit for the LCHF diet: they have an exceptional capacity to be absorbed very quickly from the stomach and converted into ketones in the liver. These fats enable the desired ketosis to be achieved significantly faster than with other fats.

Virgin coconut oil (preferably organic) is unrivaled in terms of its proportion of MCTs, with approximately 50 per cent MCT fats. When it comes to the other fats we normally use, only butter has any significant quantity of medium-chain fatty acids (approx. 10 per cent). Unfortunately, coconut oil is often classified as being unhealthy since it contains predominantly saturated fatty acids. In fact, we now know that not only is coconut fat metabolized very quickly and has a ketogenic effect, it also brings a variety of other health benefits.

OMEGA-6 FATTY ACIDS

Less favourable fats are those with a relatively high proportion of omega-6 fatty acids in comparison to omega-3 fatty acids. You should steer clear of popular oils such as safflower, wheat germ, rapeseed, soy and sunflower, not to mention any margarines produced from these oils. Unhealthy artificial trans fats can be produced from these sources, especially if they are heated: this happens during food production when hydrogen is added to liquid vegetable oils in order to make them more solid. While you should aim to include some naturally-occurring trans fats in your diet – these are the fats found in grass-fed meats and dairy – the artificial variety is damaging to health, associated with an increased risk of heart disease and cholesterol.

GOOD FATS

Omega-3 fatty acids and MCTs offer a range of benefits for the LCHF diet. You should prioritize these when selecting which fats to eat. Make organic your first choice as the healthiest option.

① FROM GRAZING ANIMALS

For all animal products, from meat to milk, the proportion of omega-3 fatty acids is highly dependent on the animal fodder: good fatty acids from fresh grass become concentrated in meat and milk. That is why it's important to focus on pasture-grazing or grass-fed animals. Lard is ideal for frying, and bacon contributes an irresistible, rounded flavour while also being rich in healthy fatty acids. Butter and cream are the only animal fats containing medium-chain fatty acids that can be swiftly converted into ketones. Both have a mellow taste and are really versatile: ideal natural flavour enhancers.

② FROM MARINE ANIMALS

High-fat sea fish, such as eel, mackerel, sardine, salmon and herring are especially rich in omega-3 fatty acids. Once again, the proportion of these nutritious fatty acids depends on the food the animals eat. Targeted, species-appropriate feeding can be used to produce very high levels of healthy fatty acids. By contrast, farmed fish that are not fed with the species' requirements in mind are relatively low in in these substances. When buying fish and shellfish caught in the wild, make sure they have been fished sustainably, as indicated by the MSC seal of approval.

③ FROM PLANT SOURCES

Two features distinguish a good vegetable oil: the ratio of omega-3 to omega-6 fatty acids and the proportion of MCTs. In cold-pressed oils all the beneficial constituents, such as vitamins, are retained. Organically produced (virgin) coconut oil should be your first choice alongside lard for frying and baking. Olive oil is primarily used for cold dishes or as a flavouring agent drizzled over food. With its high proportion of oleic acids, it regulates the fat metabolism and reduces the level of toxic fats.

The same is true for avocado oil: it consists of 50 per cent oleic acids. This oil adds a nutty element to vegetable and mushroom recipes, salads and soups. Nut oils made from walnuts, hazelnuts and macadamias are likewise suitable for cold dishes but not for cooking. These oils contain a well-balanced combination of healthy fats. Just a few drops are all that's needed to enhance salads, soups and vegetable dishes. The distinctive flavour of linseed oil also goes beautifully with these dishes, though it must not be heated. With a 6:1 ratio of omega-3 to omega-6 fatty acids, it is pretty much ideal for the human metabolism.

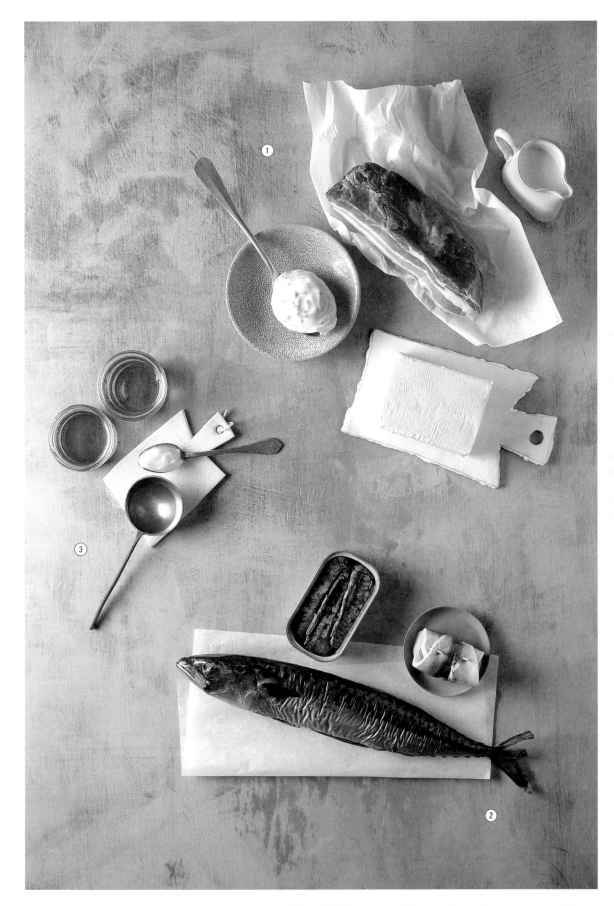

KETONES AND KETOSIS

Fat consists of a glycerol structure to which three fatty acids are coupled. When fat is broken down, these acids are released and used by our muscular system to produce energy. What is left is the glycerol component from which glucose is formed.

If fat intake is high, the body cannot utilize all the fatty acids immediately. That's why it transports any excess into the liver to be converted into so-called ketones. Ketones are acids with one particularly pertinent characteristic: they can be quickly absorbed by all cells – even in nervous tissue and in the brain. This isn't the case for fats and fatty acids because they cannot penetrate the blood-brain barrier in the form in which they are transported.

The really special thing about keto acids is that our nerve cells can use them very easily as a source of energy, which reduces the need for glucose. If sufficient ketones are available, up to 60 per cent of the brain's energy requirements can be met from this source. This also produces fewer free radicals as a potentially damaging by-product than when breaking down glucose (see page 10).

A high quantity of fat in our diet helps support brain function. Just a few weeks on a LCHF diet is almost always enough for there to be an adequate energy supply to our cells (at least for people with preexisting fat deposits). Since our hunger mechanism is constantly geared towards averting any potential energy deficit, this avoids triggering our innate alarm system and hunger is easily avoided.

DOWN WITH CARBOHYDRATES

In order to bring about these positive effects, it is essential to radically reduce your carbohydrate intake at the same time as you increase your fat intake. Only then can the right ketone concentration in the blood be achieved. On a diet with a high proportion of carbohydrates, there are practically no ketones in the blood and the brain uses glucose exclusively. Only once ketone levels rise above a value of 1 mmol/L (18 mg/dL) in the blood will ketones be used as described. This level will only be attained if carbohydrate consumption is significantly less than 100 grams (3½ ounces) per day, ideally only 50 grams (1¾ ounces).

The key to success with the LCHF diet is achieving ketosis. In this metabolic state, fat reserves are broken down without causing any hunger pangs. In this way, the brain continues to be supplied with energy even as glucose levels fall.

WHAT HAPPENS DURING KETOSIS?

Any glucose shortfall, and hence any energy deficit in the brain, inevitably leads to an intense feeling of hunger. Normally we give in to these hunger pangs and the energy deficit required to lose weight is never achieved.

But if we are able to put our bodies into ketosis, the brain never experiences this potential energy crisis and we simply don't feel hungry. Most people can then happily get by with just two meals a day. One positive side effect of this is that burning ketones results in fewer oxygen-free radicals, which can be particularly damaging to cell membranes. What's more, ketones actually strengthen the mechanisms to protect against oxidative stress and have a detoxifying impact on oxygen-free radicals.

KETONE CONCENTRATION

A good concentration of ketones in the blood should range from 1 to 3 mmol/L (18 to 54 mg/dL, see diagram on page 23). While it is possible to measure ketones in your blood, it is easier to use a urine test, which you can carry out using ketone test strips that can be found in pharmacies. When first converting to the LCHF diet, this lets you check whether your reduction in carbohydrates has been sufficient to achieve ketosis.

MEASURING KETOSIS

When you start out on the LCHF diet, measure the ketone levels in your urine each morning. The easiest and least expensive way to do this is to use a testing strip. There are many brands available in health shops or online. Whichever you buy, read the product insert in detail but usually these are the best steps to follow:

Collect urine in a clean, dry container and dip the test strip in as far as possible. Wait for 15 seconds or whatever time is stated on the brand of test strips you are using. Compare the colour on your strip to the colour array on the side of the bottle.

Any colour other than the original beige means there are some ketones in your urine. After a few days you should notice an increase in ketone concentrations in the urine. The closer the colour is toward deep purple, the more ketones there are in your body. Generally a consistent low-mid level of ketosis is the best for weight loss and feeling good.

Incorporating coconut oil, in particular, will ensure that your ketone levels rise. If this is not evident after about a week, you will need to examine your diet again for concealed carbohydrates or a high-protein intake. In which case, you may need to restrict your carbohydrate consumption further in order to reprogram your metabolism.

At the end of the 28-day plan, you should notice that the ketone concentration in your urine has reduced. This does not mean that the LCHF diet is no longer working. Quite the opposite: it indicates that your metabolism has adapted to breaking down ketones and these are now predominantly being burned and no longer excreted.

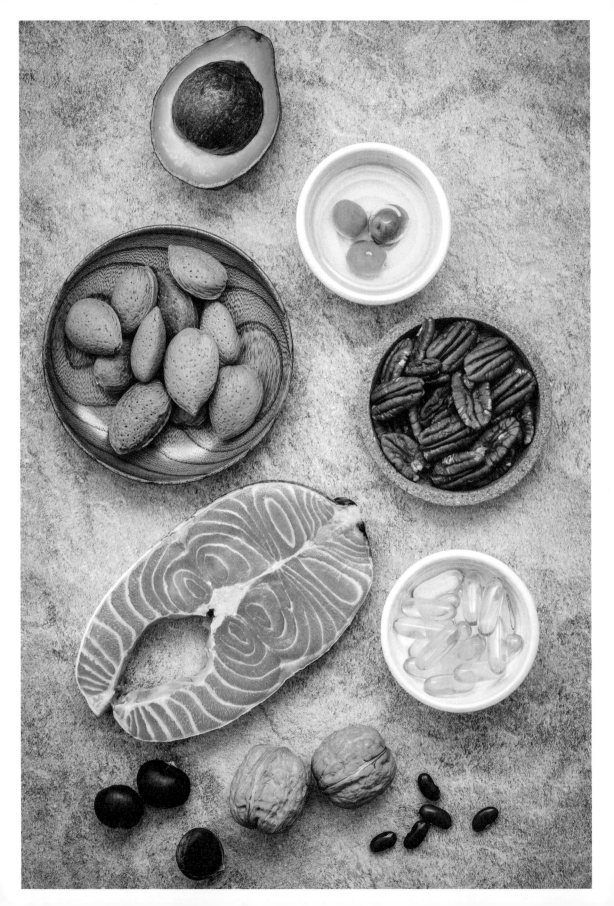

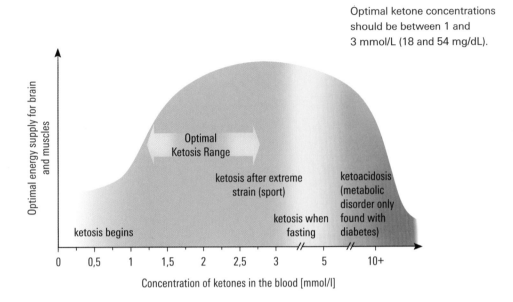

Optimal ketone concentrations should be between 1 and 3 mmol/L (18 and 54 mg/dL).

Optimal energy supply for brain and muscles

Optimal Ketosis Range

ketosis after extreme strain (sport)

ketoacidosis (metabolic disorder only found with diabetes)

ketosis when fasting

ketosis begins

0   0,5   1   1,5   2   2,5   3   5   10+

Concentration of ketones in the blood [mmol/l]

KETOSIS AND PERFORMANCE

If you can sustain ketosis in the long term, your athletic performance will also improve. Ketones provide muscles with a reliable energy supply, which means you can avoid the dreaded energy slump. This abrupt energy deficiency arises if there is a sharp drop in glucose concentration in the blood and insufficient ketones to compensate for the deficit. Ketosis also ensures a steady supply of energy to the brain, enhancing its function and making ketosis hugely significant for those suffering from dementia. Once the brain's carbohydrate metabolism can no longer operate adequately through insulin, ketones can provide the necessary energy instead.

It was established recently that Alzheimer's disease is also influenced by the same mechanism. Since insulin in the brains of those affected is no longer effective, scientists sometimes describe this form of dementia as 'type 3 diabetes'. As we know, ketones provide the brain with an alternative energy source and improve nerve function, and initial scientific research indicates significant improvements for dementia patients on a ketogenic diet.

DON'T GET YOUR TERMS CONFUSED

Ketosis is frequently confused with ketoacidosis, a life-threatening metabolic disorder found in diabetics. Ketone concentrations found in the blood of patients with this condition are ten times greater than those found in ketosis, but there is no way these kinds of ketone concentrations will be achieved purely through the LCHF diet.

1

THE 28-DAY PLAN

Welcome to the 28–day diet plan! You are going to enjoy delicious recipes every day and, as your body adapts to the new diet, you won't feel hungry or lethargic. As with any new diet, the best time to start is on a weekend so you can give yourself plenty of time to get organized. Remember to be kind to yourself and ask for support and understanding from those around you.

LOSING WEIGHT WITH THE LCHF PLAN

To lose weight with the LCHF diet, you will need to pay attention to your total calorie intake. Weigh yourself regularly for several weeks before you start the diet to check on your usual daily calorie requirement: if your weight remains constant, then your calorie intake corresponds roughly to your requirements. Check with your physician if you are unsure.

Calculating your BMI

Your Body Mass Index (BMI) is a good way to check your body fat ratio. To measure your own BMI, multiply your height in centimetres by itself. Divide your weight by this number, then times by 10,000 and round to one decimal place. An ideal ratio is around 20–25 – over 30 is considered obese. More information can be found at:
https://www.nhs.uk/live-well/healthy-weight/bmi-calculator/.

Your daily calorie requirement varies from person to person depending on your initial weight and how physically active you are. However, as a general rule, we can assume that for people with a body mass index of up to 30, reducing the daily calorie intake to approximately 1,500 calories for women and 2,000 calories for men will bring about steady weight loss. For someone with a significantly higher BMI, a higher calorie diet can still result in weight loss. On the 28-day plan, you want to ensure that your calorie intake is consistently lower than your daily calorie requirement.

With three recipes from the daily menu plan in this section you will consume roughly 1,500 calories per portion. This calorie intake can be increased, for example with smoothies or snacks, but take care to avoid the proportion of carbohydrates getting too high. Note that this book includes more great-tasting dishes than are included in the 28-day plan, giving you the inspiration to continue the LCHF diet and transform your lifestyle.

Twenty-eight days is a long time so you may not be eating all your meals at home. In restaurants, simply avoid the standard 'filling sides' such as pasta, potatoes, rice and bread. The ideal choice is some baked fish or a steak with a large salad – steer clear of the usual dressings and ask for some oil and vinegar or lemon juice. And of course, hearty portions of vegetables – preferably cooked in plenty of butter – are the perfect side dish.

SUPPLEMENTS AND ADDITIONS FOR THE 28-DAY PLAN

Top up your mineral stores

Once ketosis has been achieved, there is initially an increased excretion of minerals together with water. The best way to compensate for any potential mineral deficiencies is with meat or vegetable stock. Eat plenty of vegetables to get adequate magnesium, which is required for almost all of our body's biochemical functions. Increase your magnesium intake to start with, preferably with citrate-based supplements.

Where there is acidity....

...you need alkalinity. To keep pH values in the bloodstream constant, ketones (which are acids in terms of their chemistry) must be balanced out with appropriate alkaline substances. Vegetables and vegetable stock are good alkaline sources. If protein intake is increased at the same time, acidity levels in the blood will increase even further and consumption of alkaline foodstuffs alone will often not be sufficient to compensate. The best thing is to take alkaline, citrate-based mineral supplements (see page 30).

Bulletproof breakfast power

The perfect drink for those who refuse to eat breakfast or who are grouchy in the morning is bulletproof coffee. This is coffee enriched with butter and/or coconut oil and will fuel you with energy until midday. Not only does it fill you up, it also catapults you into the day feeling super fit. To keep things varied, why not try some cocoa with warming spices instead of coffee or tweak your coffee to suit your personal taste (see recipes on pages 170 and 171)?

Alcohol?

The good news is that alcoholic drinks are not banned. But beer is best avoided – not for nothing is it sometimes referred to as liquid bread! A glass of dry white wine is certainly permitted, likewise spirits as long as you steer clear of sweet liqueurs. Try some vodka or gin mixed with a large glass of mineral water and a dash of lime juice.

THE DAY BEFORE YOU START

The day before you start, go shopping and get everything ready in the kitchen. Clean out your fridge and store cupboard of anything you won't need. Don't buy any fast food or packaged food and prepare your first breakfast the evening before if you can, so you can take the time to enjoy it. If you are a vegetarian, or simply want to go vegetarian while on the LCHF 28-day diet plan, then substitute the meat-based recipes in the planner with any of the recipes that are marked with a 'V'. You will then need to check the calorie count for each recipe to make sure you aren't exceeding the recommended 1,500 kcal a day.

On the evening before you begin, go for a good walk outside so you can make sure to sleep well.

THE LOW-CARB HIGH-FAT KITCHEN

Good fats, meat, fish, vegetables, fruit, salads and dairy products – eating generously in all these categories will enhance the LCHF diet. The only area where you need to be careful is with foods that are rich in carbohydrates. So, clean out your store cupboard and fridge to remove any carb temptation. Make a shopping list for the first week's meals so you have everything to hand at home. And remember that buying fresh, organic produce where possible will create the healthiest and tastiest meals. As your food portions will be controlled, be generous with the quality of the ingredients.

FATS AND OILS
avocado, hemp, coconut, linseed, olive oil
butter, ghee, clarified butter
nut oils (walnut, hazelnut, macadamia nut oil)
beef tallow, animal fats (goose fat, duck fat, lard)

FISH AND SHELLFISH
eel, herring, salmon, mackerel
mussels
prawns, crab
preserved in olive oil (sardines, tuna)

MEAT AND MEAT PRODUCTS
lamb, beef, pork, game
offal (liver, kidney)
poultry, skin on (chicken, duck, goose, turkey)
rich bone broth
salami, chorizo, ham, bacon

MILK PRODUCTS
cream, quark
high-fat cheese
sheep's cheese (feta)

NUTS AND SEEDS
almonds, brazil nuts, pecans, macadamia
chia seeds, flaxseed, linseed

VEGETABLES AND SALAD
all varieties of cabbage, sauerkraut
all varieties of lettuce
artichoke
asparagus (green and white)
aubergines, courgettes
avocado
celery, cucumbers, radish
mushrooms
olives
peppers
spring onions, leek
Swiss chard, spinach
tomatoes

FRUIT
apples
apricots, plums
berries
grapefruit, oranges
lychee, papaya
pomegranate

HERBS, SPICES, SEASONINGS
all kinds of herbs
mayonnaise, aioli, béarnaise sauce
pesto
sugar-free mustard (mustard powder)
tomato purée

OTHER
dark chocolate (at least 80% cocoa solids)
eggs

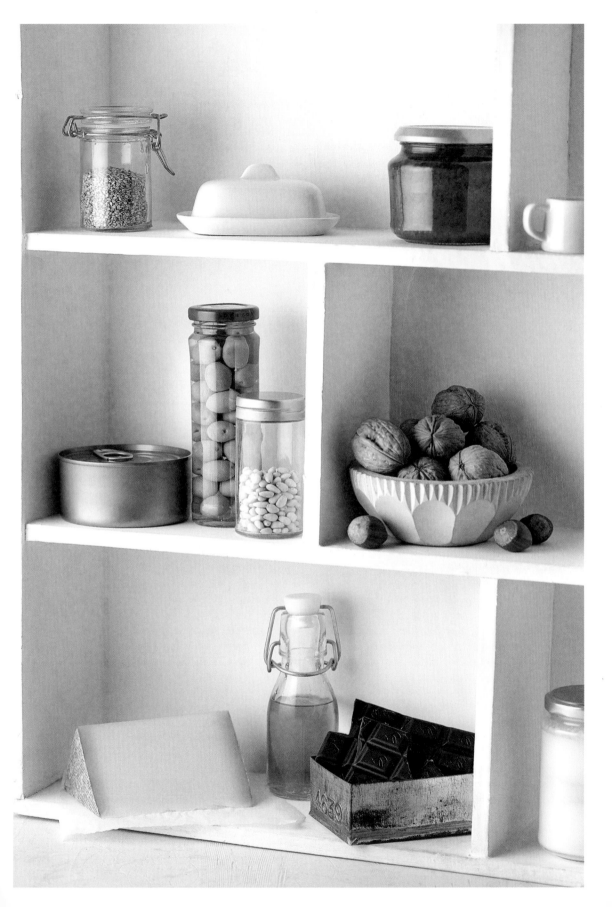

USEFUL STORECUPBOARD ADDITIONS

It's recommended you stock up on the ingredients below before you begin the 28-day LCHF plan. While some of these ingredients may sound unusual, they should all be available at your local health food shop. If you don't have them to hand, please feel free to substitute any of the specialist ingredients mentioned with locally sourced alternatives.

ACID-BASE POWDER

Ketones are acids and they accumulate in greater quantities on a LCHF diet. To keep the acid-alkaline balance in equilibrium while maintaining ketosis, an additional alkaline supplement is required. The best approach is to use an alkaline powder based on citrates, which offers protection against acidosis. These supplements are available from pharmacies or online.

AJVAR

This red pepper paste originates from the Balkans. Combining garlic, aubergine, red peppers and olive oil, it makes a delicious, low-carb condiment, provided you buy (or make) a version without too much sugar – it's best to substitute stevia instead. Ajvar is available at major supermarkets and online. You can also substitute it with sun-dried tomato.

ALMOND FLOUR

After the almonds are pressed in an oil mill, the resulting cake is finely ground, then sold as partially de-oiled almond flour. This is very low in carbohydrates and so is an ideal replacement for traditional cereal flours. The flour is also available with its natural fat content. For the recipes in this book we have used partially de-oiled almond flour. You will find it in organic and health food shops.

BIRCH SUGAR (XYLITOL)

Birch sugar, also known as xylitol, is a natural sweetener. It originally comes from birch bark but nowadays is usually manufactured synthetically. It tastes very similar to household sugar but is much more expensive. In return, however, it increases blood sugar levels significantly less than traditional sugar because only 25 per cent of its carbohydrates are broken down. Birch sugar is a good LCHF-compatible alternative to cane sugar. 1 teaspoon contains 1 kcal and no significant carbohydrate content.

CHIA SEEDS

The content of omega-3 fatty acids in chia seeds is unrivaled. They also contain large quantities of iron, magnesium, calcium, vitamins and fibre. So these little, gluten-free seeds are justifiably regarded as a superfood. They also swell easily, which makes them great as a binding agent and for baking.

COCONUT FLOUR

The flour is produced from the dried, partially de-oiled flesh of the coconut, which is then ground. It is gluten-free and its sweet coconut flavour can be used to enhance lots of dishes – either sweet or savoury. Its absorbent properties also make it ideal for thickening sauces.

COCONUT OIL

Coconut oil is particularly good for frying because it is very stable when exposed to heat. It is also great for baking. When purchasing, look for the virgin organic product. Don't confuse coconut oil with solidified coconut fat. The subtle coconut flavour of the oil gives dishes a delicate hint of coconut. If you are not so keen on the taste, instead of using the virgin oil seek out a so-called deodorized variety, where the flavourings have been removed. Coconut oil (including flavourless varieties) can be found in organic shops, health food shops and from online retailers.

COCONUT SUGAR

This sugar is ideal for the LCHF diet thanks to the minimal impact it has on blood sugar levels. It is produced from the sap of the coconut flower, which is exuded when the flower is cut.

The sugar crystals form as the substance undergoes evaporation. It can be used just like traditional sugar, it is roughly equivalent in sweetness to household sugar. It has a slightly caramel-like flavour but does not taste of coconut. 1 teaspoon of coconut sugar contains 19 kcal and 5 grams of carbohydrates.

CREAMED COCONUT
The finely grated white flesh of the coconut contains lots of oil and plant protein but few carbohydrates. It adds flavour and texture to sweet and savoury dishes. Like coconut oil, you will find it in the supermarket, at health food shops or from organic retailers. It's important to look for organic varieties here, too.

ERYTHRITOL
If a bit of sweetness is essential, this artificial sweetener is tolerated better than many other sweeteners. Erythritol contains almost no calories or carbohydrates. It is also found naturally in cheese, fruit and pistachios.

GROUND PSYLLIUM HUSKS
The finely ground husks of the psyllium seed are used as a binding and swelling agent. The powder made from the husks of the psyllium plant has practically no carbohydrates and consists of over 80 per cent dietary fibre. The recipes in this book exclusively use ready-ground psyllium husks. Substituting the same quantity of coarsely ground psyllium seed husks will not produce the same result. You can get the powder at health food shops and from organic retailers.

KETONE TEST STRIPS
These strips for measuring ketosis levels in the urine can be bought at pharmacies. They are simply dipped into the urine. Ketone levels can be determined very simply by comparing the change in colour to a comparison scale, which allows you to infer your blood ketone levels.

LIQUORICE POWDER
The sap of the liquorice root is tapped and dried, then finely ground to produce liquorice powder.

The powder is perfect for flavouring sweet or savoury dishes. You will find it at pharmacies, health food shops or online. Some people experience high blood pressure in response to liquorice. Anyone affected should speak to their physician before using it.

QUARK
A kind of curd without the added rennet or salt, quark originates from Eastern Europe. It is a soft white cheese typically described as a cross between yoghurt and cottage cheese, made by warming soured milk until it curdles. It is ideal for the LCHF diet as it is high in protein (14 grams per 100 grams) and can be high in fat (up to 40%) with negligible carbs. You can find quark online or at organic grocery and health food shops, or you can make your own.

SESAME SEED FLOUR
To make sesame seed flour, unroasted sesame seeds are de-oiled, then finely ground. It has a relatively neutral flavour and so is ideal as a flour substitute in baking. It only contains approx. 6 g carbohydrates for each 100 g (roughly equivalent to ¼ ounce per 4 ounces) and is ideal for LCHF cuisine. It can be sourced online.

STEVIA
Available in liquid or crystalline form, this extract obtained from the stevia plant is several hundred times sweeter than ordinary sugar. Due to its bitter, licorice-like aftertaste, stevia is not to everyone's liking. But it is great for a LCHF diet because it contains no calories and doesn't impact your blood sugar levels.

VANILLA POWDER
Not to be confused with vanilla sugar. To make vanilla powder the entire dried pod is finely ground. The powder is many times more intense than vanilla sugar and, most importantly, it is free from artificial additives and sugar. You will find it at pharmacies, organic groceries and health food shops.

WEEK 1

The recipes below are carefully planned to provide you with 1,500 calories a day. As each recipe indicates the calories, you may substitute for a similar recipe. Remember to cut out the sodas and too much caffeine and drink plenty of water, at least two large bottles a day. Weigh yourself to start and measure the ketone levels every morning (see page 21).

	BREAKFAST	LUNCH	SNACK	DINNER
MONDAY	Waffles with raspberry quark-style cheese (p.40)	Courgette omelette with Serrano ham (p.82)	Lemon and yoghurt jellies (p.160)	Chicken in buttermilk sauce (p.150)
TUESDAY	Almond pancakes with sour cherry compote (p.42)	Chicken nuggets with baked tomatoes (p.84)	'Quattro formaggi' muffins (p.148)	Lemon prawns on creamed spinach (p.129)
WEDNESDAY	Quark flatbread with chocolate spread (p.44)	Moussaka (p.76)	Almond and coconut cookies (p.168)	Chicken legs in bacon sauce with Savoy cabbage (p.114)
THURSDAY	White coffee smoothie (p.46)	Cheese tortillas with guacamole (p.73)	Mini peppers with cream cheese (p.152)	Meatballs with asparagus salad (p.104)
FRIDAY	Salami omelette (p.48)	Tomato and red pepper soup with Parmesan crisps (p.86)	Peanut bars (p.166)	Sea bream on green asparagus (p.130)
SATURDAY	Crunchy nut muesli (p.59)	Cheese tortillas with guacamole (p.73)	Avocado and chocolate muffins (p.163)	Pork medallions with a tomato and pepper medley (p.100)
SUNDAY	Avocado with smoked salmon mousse (p.56)	Beef soup (p.96)	Crispy courgette with herb aioli (p.146)	Ribeye steak with sauerkraut and creamy cabbage (p.117)

WEEK 2

There is a new menu of delicious recipes for you this week. The desire for carbs and sweet things can be powerful. This craving does gradually diminish, but if all else fails, you can start with adding suitable sweeteners to your food. Try gradually to reduce your reliance on sweeteners; instead reward yourself with an occasional chunk of dark chocolate. It's time for a weigh in, but don't worry if you don't see much change yet.

	BREAKFAST	LUNCH	SNACK	DINNER
MONDAY	Quark flatbread with chocolate spread (p.44)	Marinated tray-roasted summer vegetables with meatballs (p.70)	Egg carpaccio with dip (p.143)	Chicken curry with stuffed mushrooms (p.108)
TUESDAY	Bacon and quark tarte flambée (p.54)	Tuna fishcakes with cucumber salad (p.69)	Chocolate coconut balls (p.165)	Courgette lasagna with soy bolognese (p.102)
WEDNESDAY	Crackers with radish and cottage cheese (p.55)	Souvlaki kebabs with marinated feta (p.74)	Mini aubergine pizzas (p.138)	Marinated pork neck steaks with star anise (p.116)
THURSDAY	Avocado smoothie with cardamom (p.47)	Chicken nuggets with baked tomatoes (p.84)	Avocado and chocolate muffins (p.163)	Chicken in buttermilk sauce (p.105)
FRIDAY	Almond pancakes with sour cherry compote (p.42)	Cauliflower and spinach bake (p.91)	Peanut bars (p.166)	Redfish on courgette spaghetti (p.133)
SATURDAY	Salmon pancakes with spring onion dip (p.57)	Beef soup (p.96)	Mini peppers with cream cheese (p.152)	Pork tenderloin in mustard sauce with Savoy cabbage and mushrooms (p.113)
SUNDAY	Waffles with raspberry quark-style cheese (p.40)	Sauerkraut and bacon patties (p.90)	Almond and coconut cookies (p.168)	Duck breast on a bed of chicory (p.123)

WEEK 3

By now your cravings should have diminished, so you can look to increase your exercise and activity. A good daily walk is a minimum, but pick up the pace if you can with something you enjoy – yoga, swimming or cycling are all good. You should see a weight reduction by now. Remember to keep up the fluid intake.

	BREAKFAST	LUNCH	SNACK	DINNER
MONDAY	Crunchy nut muesli (p.59)	Courgette omelette with Serrano ham (p.82)	Eggs baked in tomatoes (p.143)	Halloumi with a papaya and tomato salsa (p.124)
TUESDAY	Avocado with smoked salmon mousse (p.56)	Veggie spaghetti with mushroom sauce (p.88)	Parmesan and courgette patties with red pesto (p.141)	Monkfish in an orange and pepper sauce (p.134)
WEDNESDAY	Salami omelette (p.48)	Chicken nuggets with baked tomatoes (p.84)	Almond and coconut cookies (p.168)	Meatballs with asparagus salad (p.104)
THURSDAY	Cream cheese smoothie with strawberries (p.46)	Sauerkraut and bacon patties (p.90)	Spinach muffins with bacon (p.150)	Pork medallions with a tomato and pepper medley (p.100)
FRIDAY	Coconut pancakes with blueberry yoghurt (p.43)	Tuna fishcakes with cucumber salad (p.69)	Yoghurt panna cotta with strawberry sauce (p.157)	Courgette lasagna with soy bolognese (p.102)
SATURDAY	Waffles with raspberry quark-style cheese (p.40)	Souvlaki kebabs with marinated feta (p.74)	Crispy courgette with herb aioli (p.146)	Ribeye steak with sauerkraut and creamy cabbage (p.117)
SUNDAY	Cottage cheese flatbread (p.61)	Moussaka (p.76)	'Quattro formaggi' muffins (p.148)	Lamb fillet with a parsley and mustard topping (p.110)

WEEK 4

Well done for making it to the last week. You should be feeling lighter, more energized and more focused. You don't need to stop the diet after this week. Now you have the recipes under your belt and plenty more in the book to explore, go ahead and enjoy cooking and eating more LCHF meals.

	BREAKFAST	LUNCH	SNACK	DINNER
MONDAY	Almond pancakes with sour cherry compote (p.42)	Cheese tortillas with guacamole (p.82)	Stuffed eggs with bacon (p.142)	Marinated pork neck steaks with star anise (p.116)
TUESDAY	Quark flatbread with chocolate spread (p.44)	Marinated tray-roasted summer vegetables with meatballs (p.70)	Lemon and yoghurt jellies (p.160)	Cauliflower risotto (p.126)
WEDNESDAY	Salmon pancakes with spring onion dip (p.57)	Cauliflower and spinach bake (p.91)	Peanut bars (p.166)	Chicken in creamy curry sauce with stuffed mushrooms (p.108)
THURSDAY	Blueberry and liquorice smoothie (p.47)	Tomato and red pepper soup with Parmesan crisps (p.152)	Chocolate coconut balls (p.165)	Chicken in buttermilk sauce (p.105)
FRIDAY	Waffles with raspberry quark-style cheese (p.41)	Moussaka (p.76)	Parmesan and courgette patties with red pesto (p.141)	Lemon prawns on creamed spinach (p.129)
SATURDAY	Crunchy nut muesli (p.59)	Chicken nuggets with baked tomatoes (p.84)	Mini aubergine pizzas (p.138)	Lamb fillet with a parsley and mustard topping (p.110)
SUNDAY	Bacon and quark tarte flambée (p.54)	Cauliflower and turmeric cheese fritters (p.85)	Choco-nut bites (p.164)	Pork tenderloin in mustard sauce with Savoy cabbage and mushrooms (p.113)

2

BREAKFAST

Sweet or savory is not so important,
but getting the day off to a keto start is
crucial. Try simple standbys or quick dishes,
like scrambled eggs or fruit salad.
To make sure you have time for a substantial
breakfast, lots of the preparation can be
done the night before.

ORANGE AND CHIA
CREAM WITH PISTACHIOS

zest and juice of 1 orange
3 medium eggs
100 g (scant ½ cup) cream
1 tablespoon chia seeds, plus extra for
  scattering
100 g (1⅓ cup) shelled pistachios
  (roasted, unsalted)

Serves 2
Preparation: approx. 20 minutes
Per portion: approx. 480 kcal, 19 g
protein, 39 g fat, 10 g carbohydrate

Choose a pan that is large enough to form a bain-marie, fill with 1 cm (½ inch) of water and bring to the boil.

Meanwhile, measure 100 ml (scant ½ cup) of the orange juice and mix this with the orange zest, eggs and cream in a heatproof bowl (metal, if possible) until smooth. Heat the mixture over the bain-marie, stirring constantly, for 5–6 minutes until it has thickened.

Stir in the chia seeds and stand the bowl in cold water to chill for 10 minutes to prevent it cooking any further. Stir the cream occasionally as it cools.

Divide the cream between two little bowls and serve scattered with pistachios and chia seeds.

PREPARE THE NIGHT BEFORE
This creamy dish is great prepared ahead of time. In fact, after chilling overnight in the fridge the consistency will be even creamier. The following morning, just scatter over the pistachios and chia seeds and it's ready to enjoy.

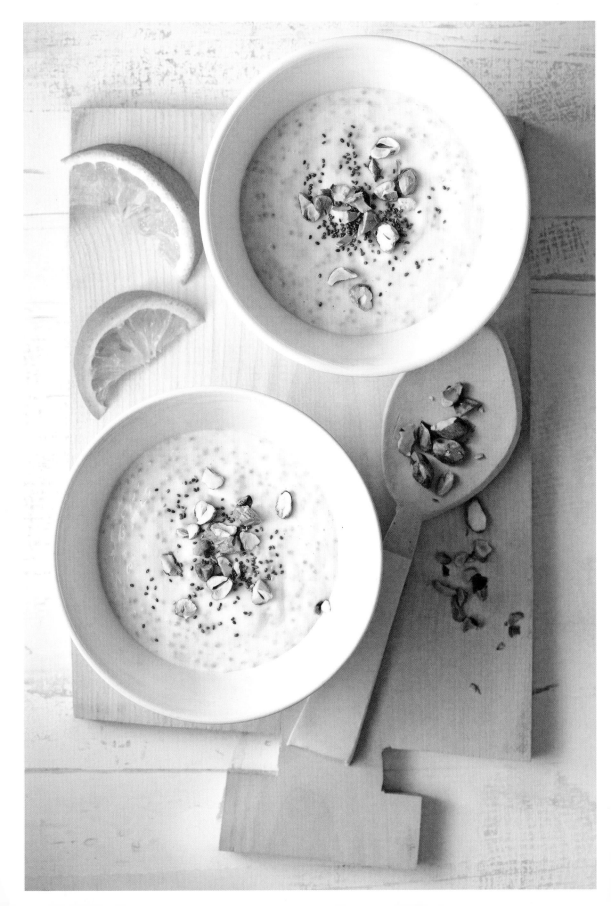

WAFFLES WITH
RASPBERRY QUARK-STYLE CHEESE

(V)

FOR THE WAFFLES
3 medium eggs
75 g (⅓ cup) cream
3 tablespoons ground psyllium husks
salt
soft butter, for greasing

FOR THE QUARK
50 g (scant ½ cup) raspberries, plus
    extra to serve
200 g (heaping ¾ cup) quark
    (40% fat)
3 tablespoons Greek yoghurt

Serves: 2
Preparation: approx. 25 minutes
Per portion: approx. 435 kcal, 23 g
protein, 34 g fat, 7 g carbohydrate

Stir the eggs, cream, ground psyllium husks, a pinch of salt and 150 ml (⅔ cup) cold water with a whisk until you have a smooth batter. Leave the batter to stand for 5 minutes.

Meanwhile, crush the raspberries slightly in a bowl using a fork. Add the quark and yoghurt and stir together until creamy.

Heat the waffle iron to medium, then use a pastry brush to apply a thin layer of butter over the surface. Put a quarter of the batter into the waffle maker, close and cook for 3–4 minutes until light golden brown and crisp. Transfer to a plate, cover and keep warm. Make three more waffles in the same way with the remaining batter. Arrange on two plates and serve with the quark and a few extra raspberries.

NO WAFFLE MAKER?

No worries, the batter can also be used to make pancakes. To do this, melt 1 tablespoon of butter in a large, non-stick pan over a medium heat. For one small pancake, add 1 tablespoon of batter and cook for 2 minutes, then flip it over using a spatula and cook for 2 minutes on the other side. The batter will make roughly eight small pancakes, which go just as well with the raspberry quark as the waffles.

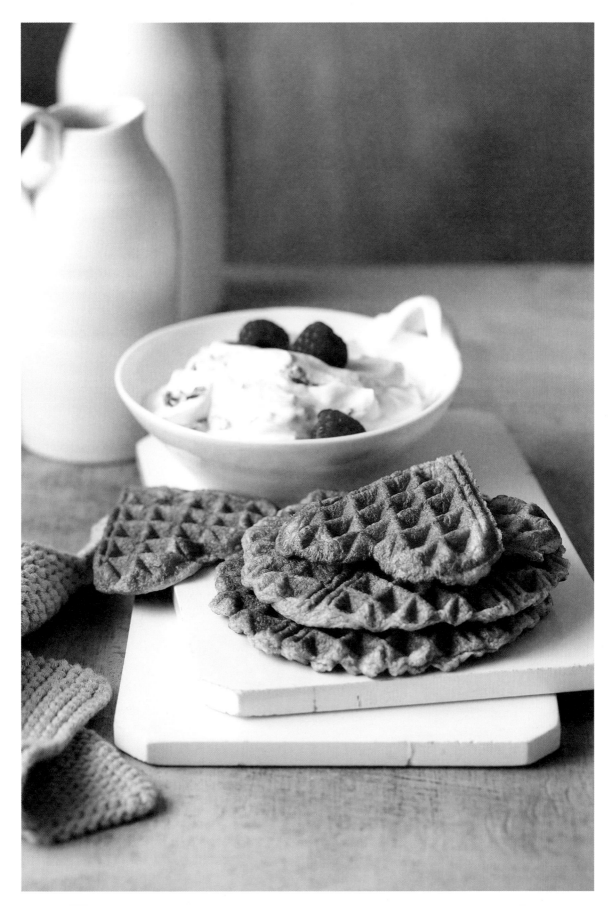

ALMOND PANCAKES
WITH SOUR CHERRY COMPOTE

(V)

FOR THE PANCAKES
3 medium eggs
50 g (¼ cup) cream
1 tablespoon almond butter
50 g (½ cup) ground almonds
1 tablespoon ground psyllium husks
½ teaspoon vanilla powder
3 tablespoons coconut oil

FOR THE COMPOTE
100 g (⅔ cup) sour cherries (or defrosted
    frozen sour cherries)
1 tablespoon lemon juice
½ teaspoon ground cardamom
½ teaspoon ground cinnamon
1 tablespoon chia seeds

Serves: 2
Preparation: approx. 15 minutes
Standing time: approx. 10 minutes
Per portion: approx. 600 kcal, 19 g
protein, 53 g fat, 10 g carbohydrate

To make the pancakes, put the eggs, cream, almond butter, ground almonds, ground psyllium husks and vanilla powder into a bowl with 100 ml (scant ½ cup) water and whisk swiftly to create a smooth batter. Let the batter stand for 10 minutes.

Meanwhile, put the sour cherries into a pan with the lemon juice and 1 tablespoon of water, bring briefly to the boil, then remove from the heat. Stir in the cardamom, cinnamon and chia seeds and let it stand for about 10 minutes.

Heat the coconut oil in a large non-stick frying pan. Add 1–2 tablespoons of batter to the pan for each pancake and cook over a medium heat for 1–2 minutes until golden brown underneath. Flip over and continue cooking on the other side for 1–2 minutes until golden.

Make a total of eight pancakes, arrange on two plates and serve with the cherry compote.

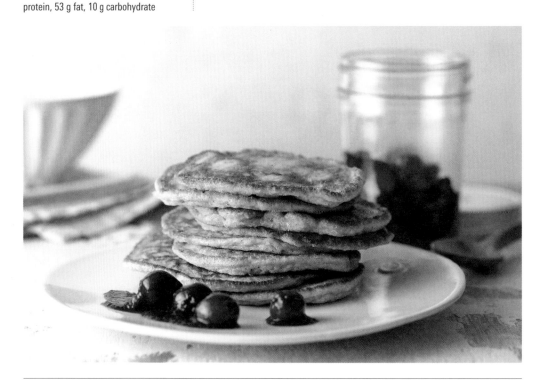

COCONUT PANCAKES
WITH BLUEBERRY YOGHURT

(V)

FOR THE PANCAKES
3 medium eggs
80 g (⅓ cup) crème fraîche
2 tablespoons desiccated coconut
2 teaspoons ground psyllium husks
3 tablespoons coconut oil

FOR THE YOGHURT
50 g (⅓ cup) blueberries
200 g (1½ cups) yoghurt
1 tablespoon creamed coconut
½ teaspoon vanilla powder
birch sugar (xylitol, optional)

Serves: 2
Preparation: approx. 25 minutes
Standing time: approx. 10 minutes
Per portion: approx. 635 kcal, 16 g
protein, 59 g fat, 9 g carbohydrate

Briskly whisk together the eggs, crème fraîche, desiccated coconut and ground psyllium husks to create a smooth batter. Let it stand for about 10 minutes.

Meanwhile, mash the blueberries slightly with a fork. Add the yoghurt, creamed coconut and vanilla powder and stir. If desired, adjust to taste with some birch sugar. Transfer to the fridge.

Heat the coconut oil in a large non-stick frying pan. Use 1–2 tablespoons of batter per pancake and cook, covered, over a medium heat for roughly 2 minutes until golden brown. Flip them over and continue cooking on the other side for 1–2 minutes until golden.

Make a total of eight pancakes, arrange them between two plates and serve with the blueberry yoghurt.

WARM OR COLD
Everyone has their own preference. These pancakes can easily be prepared the previous evening and still taste great cold the following morning. If that doesn't appeal, you can either cook them fresh in the morning or briefly reheat them in the microwave or oven.

QUARK FLATBREAD
WITH CHOCOLATE SPREAD

(v)

FOR THE QUARK FLATBREADS
100 g (⅓ cup) quark
    (40% fat)
2 medium eggs, separated
2 tablespoons almond flour
1 teaspoon ground psyllium husks
salt

FOR THE CHOCOLATE SPREAD
1 avocado
1 tablespoon cream
1 tablespoon cocoa powder
birch sugar (xylitol, optional)

Serves 2
Preparation: approx. 20 minutes
Baking: approx. 30 minutes
Per portion: approx. 475 kcal, 25 g
protein, 39 g fat, 4 g carbohydrate

Preheat the oven to 150°C (300°F). Line a baking tray with greaseproof paper. Squeeze the quark thoroughly in a clean tea towel to remove as much moisture as possible. Whisk the egg whites with a pinch of salt until stiff. Quickly stir together the quark, egg yolks, almond flour and ground psyllium husks. Carefully fold in the whisked egg whites.

Use a tablespoon to create four equal dollops of quark mixture on the baking tray and press slightly flat. Bake in the centre of the oven for 25–30 minutes. Turn off the oven and allow the breads to cool inside. Leave to cool in the oven.

Meanwhile, prepare the chocolate spread. To do this, halve the avocado, remove the stone and scoop out the flesh. Transfer to a blender along with the cream, cocoa powder and, if desired, the birch sugar. Blend to a purée.

Serve the cooled quark flatbreads on two plates, topped with the chocolate spread.

QUARK ROLLS

These protein-rich quark flatbreads also make a great alternative to bread rolls. Since they have neither a sweet nor savoury flavour themselves, they taste just as delicious with slightly sweet toppings and spreads (such as the chocolate spread here) or with savoury toppings, such as a slice of sausage or cheese.

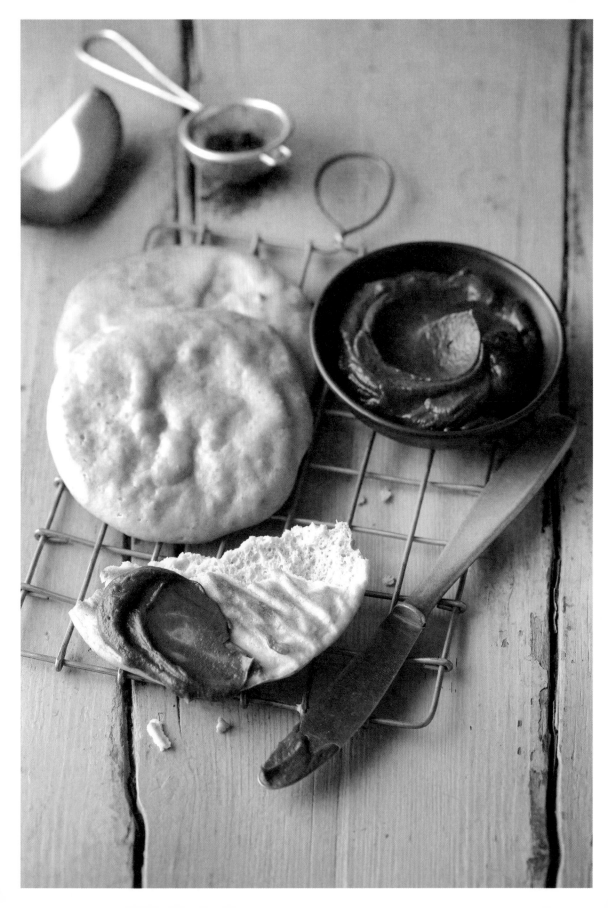

WHITE COFFEE
SMOOTHIE

150 ml (⅔ cup) cold coffee
150 ml (⅔ cup) almond milk
    (unsweetened)
100 g (⅓ cup) soured cream
50 g (⅓ cup) blanched almonds
1 tablespoon creamed coconut
3 medium eggs
½ teaspoon vanilla powder
birch sugar (xylitol, optional)
4 ice cubes
cocoa powder, for decorating

Serves 2
Preparation: approx. 10 minutes
Per portion: approx. 490 kcal, 18 g
protein, 43 g fat, 9 g carbohydrate

Put the coffee into a blender along with the almond milk, soured cream, almonds, creamed coconut, eggs and vanilla powder. Blend until the almonds are finely ground and all the ingredients are thoroughly combined. If desired, adjust to taste with some birch sugar.

Add two ice cubes each to two large glasses and pour over the coffee smoothie. Top with a dusting of cocoa powder and serve immediately.

CREAM CHEESE SMOOTHIE
WITH STRAWBERRIES

150 g (1 cup) strawberries, hulled
140 g (heaping ½ cup) full-fat
    cream cheese
180 g (¾ cup) coconut milk (tinned)
2 medium eggs
½ teaspoon vanilla powder
birch sugar (xylitol, optional)

Serves 2
Preparation: approx. 15 minutes
Per portion: approx. 465 kcal,
14 g protein, 41 g fat, 8 g carbohydrate

Depending on how large they are, halve or quarter the strawberries. Set aside four strawberry halves for decoration.

Put the remaining strawberries into a blender with the cream cheese, coconut milk, eggs and vanilla powder and blend until smooth. If desired, adjust to taste with some birch sugar.

Pour the smoothie into two large glasses, decorate with the halved strawberries and serve.

AVOCADO SMOOTHIE
WITH CARDAMOM

(V)

1 avocado, halved and destoned
2 medium eggs
100 g (scant ½ cup) coconut milk
   (tinned)
50 g (¼ cup) cream
½ teaspoon vanilla powder
½ teaspoon ground cardamom
100 g (¾ cup) raspberries
birch sugar (xylitol, optional)
6 ice cubes

Serves 2
Preparation: approx. 15 minutes
Per portion: approx. 525 kcal,
12 g protein, 50 g fat, 5 g carbohydrate

Put the avocado flesh into a blender and add the eggs, coconut milk, cream, vanilla powder, cardamom and raspberries (reserving four of the best for decoration) and blend until smooth. Add 100–150 ml (½–⅓ cup) water depending on the desired consistency and blend the smoothie again. If desired, adjust to taste with some birch sugar.

Put three ice cubes each into two large glasses and pour over the smoothie. Decorate with the reserved raspberries and serve.

BLUEBERRY AND
LIQUORICE SMOOTHIE

150 g (1 cup) blueberries
300 g (1¼ cup) soured cream
150 g (½ cup) Greek yoghurt
3 tablespoons creamed coconut
1 teaspoon liquorice powder
1 teaspoon vanilla powder
birch sugar (xylitol, optional)

Serves 2
Preparation: approx. 10 minutes
Per portion: approx. 630 kcal,
9 g protein, 58 g fat, 16 g carbohydrate

Set aside four of the best blueberries for decoration. Add the remaining blueberries to a blender along with the soured cream, yoghurt, creamed coconut, liquorice powder and vanilla powder and blend until smooth. If desired, adjust to taste with some birch sugar.

Transfer into two large glasses, decorate with the reserved blueberries and serve.

SALAMI OMELETTE

50 g (1¾ oz) Gouda (or other hard
   cheese), roughly grated
50 g (1¾ oz) Parmesan, roughly grated
3 medium eggs
2 tablespoons cream
2 teaspoons butter
6 slices of salami
4 chives, cut into little pieces
2 sprigs of coriander
salt and pepper

Serves 2
Preparation: approx. 25 minutes
Per portion: approx. 400 kcal,
29 g protein, 31 g fat, 1 g carbohydrate

Mix the Gouda and Parmesan well. Beat the eggs and cream
with a fork and season with salt and pepper.

Melt 1 teaspoon of the butter in a non-stick pan over a medium
heat. Spread half the cheese mixture evenly over the pan, cover
and let the cheese melt for 1 minute.

Pour half the egg mixture over the cheese, distributing it evenly
by swirling the pan. Cover the pan and cook over a medium heat
for 2 minutes.

Cover one half of the omelette with three slices of salami and
carefully fold over the other half of the omelette using a spatula.
Cover the pan again and continue cooking the omelette for
2 minutes. Flip the omelette and cook the other side for another
2 minutes until the egg mixture has completely set.

Slip the omelette onto a plate and cover with foil to keep warm.
Cook a second omelette from the remaining ingredients. Scatter
chopped chives over both omelettes and garnish with coriander
to serve.

A RANGE OF FILLINGS

Use these ingredients as fillings to ensure you get plenty of
variety at the breakfast table: different hard cheeses such as
Monterey Jack or Edam, which give similar results to Gouda;
finely chopped vegetables such as cherry tomatoes, shallots,
red onions or pepper. Add in some aromatic fresh herbs such
as basil, oregano, flat-leaf parsley, thyme or sage. Is there some
leftover smoked ham lurking in your fridge? Or maybe some
Parma ham or smoked turkey breast or even some bacon?
Fantastic, just toss it into the omelette!

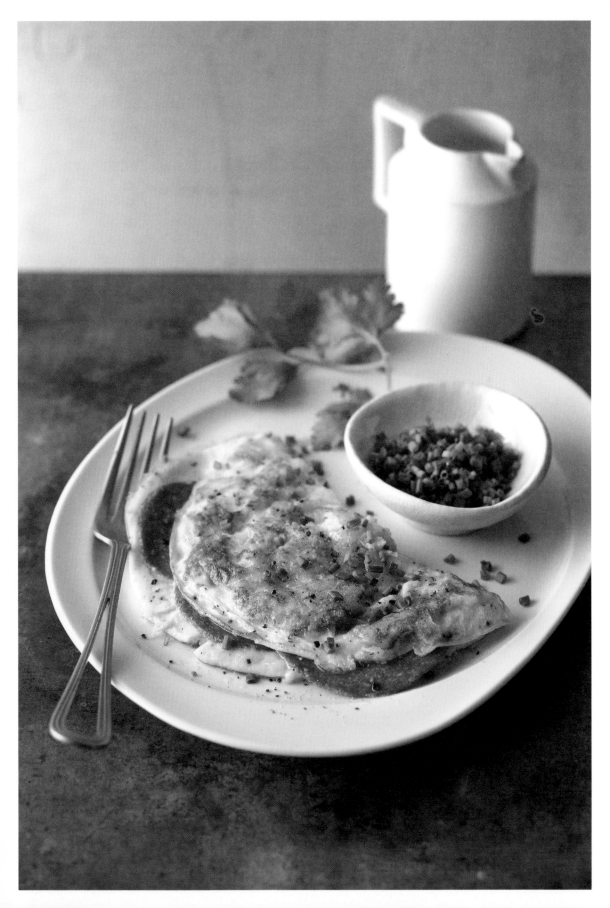

GOUDA, TOMATO AND HAM OMELETTE

4 medium eggs
2½ tablespoons cream
8 teaspoons butter
2 tomatoes, cut into roughly 5-mm
    (¼-inch) thick slices
40 g (1½ oz) Gouda, roughly grated
2 slices of cooked ham, finely chopped
salt and pepper

Serves 2
Preparation: approx. 15 minutes
Per portion: approx. 495 kcal,
31 g protein, 40 g fat, 3 g carbohydrate

Whisk the eggs into the cream until smooth and season with salt and pepper. Melt 4 teaspoons of the butter in a non-stick pan over a medium heat. Add half the egg mixture and tilt the pan to distribute evenly. Cover the pan and cook the egg mixture for 2 minutes.

Cover one half of the omelette with half the sliced tomato, cheese and ham. Carefully fold over the other half of the omelette using a spatula. Return the lid to the pan and continue cooking for 1 minute. Turn the omelette and cook the other side for 1 minute, until the egg mixture has set completely and the cheese inside has melted.

Slide the filled omelette onto a plate and cover with foil to keep warm. Make a second omelette in the same way from the remaining ingredients and serve.

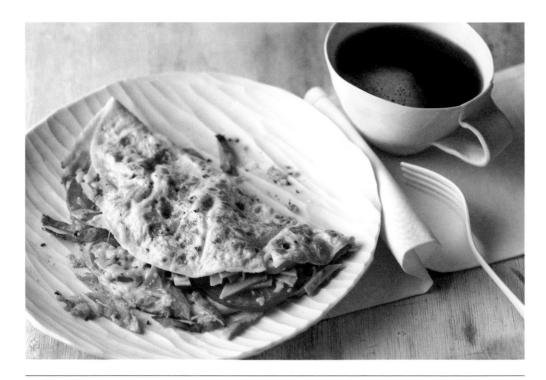

SPINACH AND BLUE CHEESE OMELETTE

(V)

150 g (5 oz) fresh or frozen spinach, defrosted
4 medium eggs
2½ tablespoons cream
freshly grated nutmeg
2 teaspoons butter
80 g (3 oz) blue cheese
salt and pepper

Serves 2
Preparation: approx. 15 minutes
Per portion: approx. 435 kcal,
21 g protein, 38 g fat, 2 g carbohydrate

Add the spinach to a blender with the eggs, cream, salt, pepper and nutmeg and blend until smooth.

Melt 1 teaspoon of the butter in a non-stick pan over a medium heat. Add half the egg mixture and tilt the pan to distribute evenly. Cover the pan and cook for 2 minutes.

Crumble half the blue cheese over one half of the omelette. Carefully fold over the other half of the omelette using a spatula, cover and continue cooking for 1 minute. Flip the omelette over, cover and cook the other side for 1 minute until the spinach mixture has set and the cheese inside has melted.

Slip the omelette onto a plate and cover with foil to keep warm. Make the second omelette in the same way from the remaining ingredients and serve.

OVEN-BAKED OMELETTE WITH CREAMED MUSHROOMS

4 medium eggs
150 g (⅔ cup) cream
3 sprigs of parsley, finely chopped
    (or 1 tablespoon frozen chopped
    parsley)
freshly grated nutmeg
1 teaspoon butter
150 g (2 ¾ cups) chanterelles (or other
    mushrooms), large ones halved or
    quartered
3 slices of cooked ham, diced
salt and pepper

Serves 2
Preparation: approx. 20 minutes
Per portion: approx. 455 kcal,
23 g protein, 39 g fat, 3 g carbohydrate

Line a high-sided baking tray up to the rim with greaseproof paper. Preheat the oven to 200°C (400°F).

Whisk together the eggs, 100 g (scant ½ cup) of the cream and the chopped parsley until smooth. Season with salt, pepper and nutmeg. Pour the egg mixture over the baking tray and tilt the tray to spread it out evenly. Place the tray in the centre of the oven and bake for 10 minutes until the egg mixture has set completely and has started to brown slightly.

Meanwhile, melt the butter in a pan over a high heat and sauté the mushrooms for 2 minutes. Add the diced ham and continue cooking everything for a further 1 minute.

Pour in the remaining cream, bring to the boil and simmer for 1 minute until it has reduced to a thick and creamy sauce. Season to taste with more salt, pepper and nutmeg.

Remove the omelette from the oven and use the greaseproof paper to transfer it to a chopping board. Use a spatula to help release it from the greaseproof paper and roll it up. Slice diagonally into six equal pieces, transfer onto two plates and serve with the creamy chanterelle mushrooms.

MIX IT UP

You can use other types of mushroom instead of the chanterelles. Button mushrooms, king oyster mushrooms, shiitake and Chinese mushrooms are available all year round. Or maybe you've gone out mushroom picking and gathered a good haul yourself; in which case, you can use this recipe to rustle up something truly delicious from your basket.

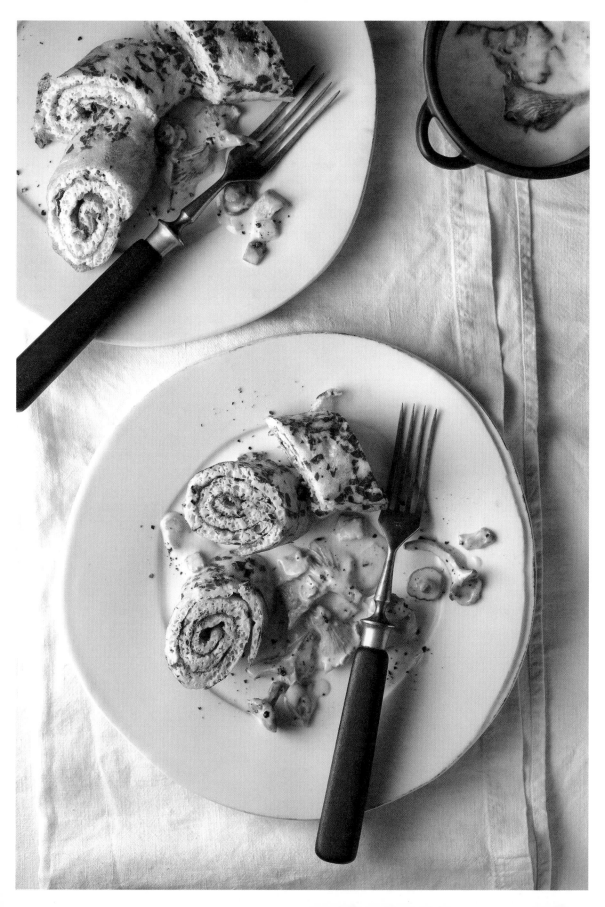

BACON AND
QUARK TARTE FLAMBÉE

100 g (⅓ cup) quark (20% fat)
2 medium eggs
1 tablespoon coconut flour
150 g (5 oz) Gouda, roughly grated
2 spring onions, finely sliced
5 rashers bacon, finely chopped
80 g (⅓ cup) crème fraîche
salt

Serves 2
Preparation: approx. 20 minutes
Baking: approx. 35 minutes
Per portion: approx. 585 kcal,
40 g protein, 45 g fat, 4 g carbohydrate

Preheat the oven to 170°C (350°F). Line a baking tray with greaseproof paper. Stir together the quark, eggs, coconut flour, a pinch of salt and a third of the Gouda. Transfer to the baking tray and spread the mixture out to create a square with 20 cm (7 inch) sides. Slide the tray into the centre of the oven and bake for 15 minutes.

Remove the baking tray from the oven (but leave the oven on), spread the quark base with crème fraîche and scatter over the bacon, spring onions and remaining cheese.

Return to the oven to cook for a further 15–20 minutes until the cheese is nicely golden. Remove, slice into quarters and serve on two plates.

A TASTY ALTERNATIVE
Try using red, yellow or green peppers sliced into thin strips, little precooked broccoli florets or sliced mushrooms.

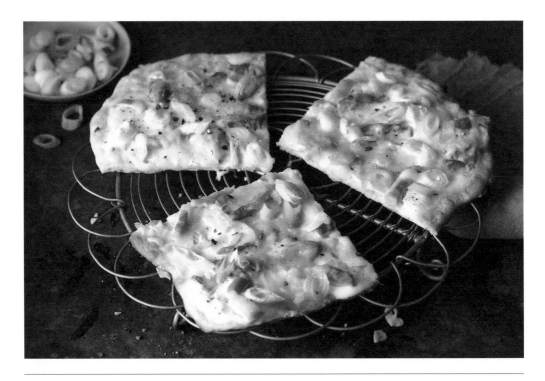

CRACKERS WITH RADISH
AND COTTAGE CHEESE

(V)

FOR THE CRACKERS

80 g (½ cup) linseeds, whole

1 medium egg

50 g (1¾ oz) Gouda, roughly grated

1 tablespoon sesame seeds

1 tablespoon sunflower seeds

salt and pepper

FOR THE COTTAGE CHEESE

6 radishes, roughly grated

2 sprigs of fresh dill, leaves finely
    chopped (or 1 teaspoon chopped
    frozen dill)

200 g (heaping ¾ cup) cottage cheese

salt and pepper

Serves 2

Preparation: approx. 20 minutes

Baking: approx. 25 minutes

Per portion: approx. 485 kcal,

38 g protein, 31 g fat, 5 g carbohydrate

Whisk the linseeds into the egg and 2 tablespoons of lukewarm water then let it stand for 15 minutes. Preheat the oven to 150°C (300°F). Line a baking tray with greaseproof paper.

Meanwhile, add the Gouda to the soaked linseed together with the sesame and sunflower seeds and stir well. Season with a pinch of salt and pepper.

Use a tablespoon to scoop eight equal-size portions of the mixture onto the baking tray, spacing them well apart. Press the dollops of mixture flat. Put the tray into the centre of the oven and bake the crackers for a total of 25 minutes, turning once after 15 minutes.

Stir the radishes and dill into the cottage cheese and season to taste with salt and pepper.

Once the crackers are cooked, remove them from the oven and use the greaseproof paper to transfer them to a wire rack to cool completely. Arrange on two plates with the radish and cottage cheese to serve.

AVOCADO WITH SMOKED
SALMON MOUSSE

150 g (5 oz) smoked salmon, chopped
    into small chunks
zest and juice of ½ lemon
50 g (¼ cup) full-fat cream cheese
80 g (⅓ cup) Greek yoghurt
pinch of ground psyllium husks
4 sprigs of dill, leaves finely chopped (or
    1 tablespoon chopped frozen dill)
1 avocado, peeled and destoned
salt and pepper

Serves 2
Preparation: approx. 20 minutes
Per portion: approx. 490 kcal,
19 g protein, 44 g fat, 3 g carbohydrate

Put the salmon into a blender or food processor. Add 1 tablespoon of the lemon juice with the lemon zest, cream cheese, yoghurt, ground psyllium husks and dill and blend everything until smooth. Season to taste with salt and pepper. Chill the salmon mousse for 5 minutes.

Slice the avocado halves lengthways into roughly 4-mm (⅛-inch) thick slices and arrange these in a fan pattern on two plates. Drizzle or brush the cut surfaces with the remaining lemon juice to prevent them from going brown.

Using a damp spoon, scoop up little mounds of salmon mousse and arrange these on the plates next to the avocado to serve.

SALMON PANCAKES
WITH SPRING ONION DIP

FOR THE PANCAKES

100 g (3½ oz) smoked salmon, roughly
    chopped
juice of ¼ lemon
2 medium eggs
30 g (2 tablespoons) cream
2 sprigs of dill, leaves picked
1 tablespoon ground psyllium husks
3 teaspoons coconut oil
salt and pepper

FOR THE DIP

3 spring onions, sliced diagonally
1 tablespoon mayonnaise
50 g (¼ cup) soured cream
½ teaspoon mild ground paprika
salt and pepper

Serves 2
Preparation: approx. 25 minutes
Per portion: approx. 390 kcal,
18 g protein, 34 g fat, 3 g carbohydrate

Put the salmon, lemon juice, eggs, cream and dill in a blender and process until smooth. Quickly fold in the ground psyllium husks, season to taste with salt and pepper and let it stand for 10 minutes.

Meanwhile, stir the spring onions into the mayonnaise, soured cream and ground paprika. Season to taste with salt and pepper.

Melt the coconut oil in a non-stick pan over a medium heat. Make four pancakes, each using 1½ tablespoons of the mixture and cook each side for 2–3 minutes. Transfer the salmon pancakes to a plate and serve with the dip.

CUCUMBER SALAD

Transform the dip into a cucumber salad, which also goes beautifully with the smoked salmon pancakes. Replace the spring onion with ½ cucumber, peeled and thinly sliced, and add 1 tablespoon white wine vinegar: your speedy cucumber salad is ready.

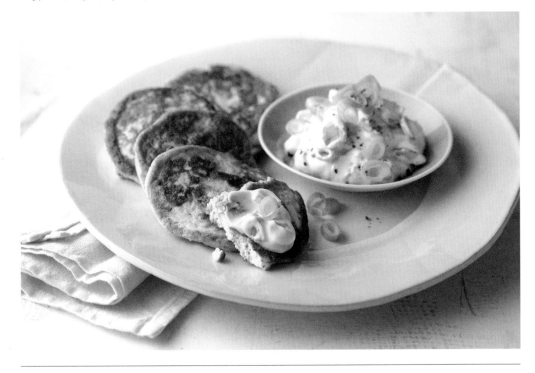

RICH ALMOND BREAD

coconut oil, for greasing
250 g (scant 1 cup) Greek yoghurt
6 medium eggs
40 g (¼ cup) ground linseed
50 g (scant ½ cup) sunflower seeds
120 g (1¼ cup) ground almonds
2 tablespoons ground psyllium husks
2 teaspoons baking powder
salt

Makes 1 loaf (roughly 15 slices)
Preparation: approx. 15 minutes
Baking: approx. 45 minutes
Per slice: approx. 130 kcal, 6 g protein,
11 g fat, 2 g carbohydrate

Preheat the oven to 180°C (350°F). Grease a loaf tin with coconut oil. Mix the yoghurt, eggs and a pinch of salt in a bowl. Then add the linseed, sunflower seeds and almonds and stir well.

Finally, add the ground psyllium husks and baking powder and fold in swiftly using a whisk. Leave the dough to prove for 10 minutes, then transfer to the greased loaf tin and bake in the centre of the oven for 45 minutes.

Remove, let it cool briefly, then carefully turn the bread out of the tin. Leave to cool completely on a wire rack.

SPICE IT UP

Give the loaf an unmistakable flavour and create endless different versions. Great options include fennel seeds, caraway, dried thyme or rosemary: 1 teaspoon will suffice in each case. A dash of red wine vinegar gives the bread a pleasant acidity.

CRUNCHY NUT MUESLI

FOR THE MUESLI
2 tablespoons hazelnuts
1 tablespoon salted peanuts
1 tablespoon flaked almonds
1 tablespoon coconut flakes
1 tablespoon pumpkin seeds
1 tablespoon sunflower seeds
1 teaspoon coconut oil
pinch of ground cinnamon
½ teaspoon ground cardamom

FOR THE QUARK
200 g (heaping ¾ cup) quark
    (20% fat)
½ teaspoon vanilla powder
birch sugar (xylitol, optional)

Serves 2
Preparation: approx. 15 minutes
Baking: approx. 10 minutes
Per portion: approx. 445 kcal, 22 g
protein, 36 g fat, 8 g carbohydrate

Preheat the oven to 160°C (325°F). Line a baking tray with greaseproof paper. Roughly chop the hazelnuts and peanuts. Add to a bowl with the flaked almonds, coconut flakes, pumpkin seeds and sunflower seeds. Add the coconut oil, cinnamon and cardamom and combine everything well using your hands.

Spread evenly over the baking tray and place in the centre of the oven. Don't put too much to bake on the tray, otherwise you won't get a crunchy muesli. Bake for 8–10 minutes. Stir the mixture halfway through to ensure the nuts and seeds toast evenly.

Meanwhile, stir the quark and vanilla powder together until smooth. If desired, adjust to taste with some birch sugar. Divide the quark between two bowls. Remove the muesli from the oven, leave to cool slightly, sprinkle over the quark and serve.

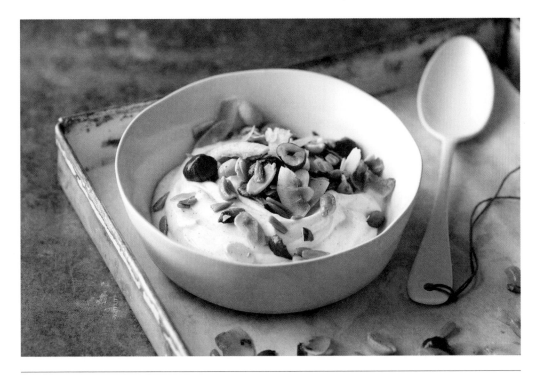

LINSEED CRISPBREADS

1 medium egg
100 g (⅔ cup) ground linseed
2 tablespoons almond flour
salt

Makes 10
Preparation: approx. 15 minutes
Standing time: approx. 10 minutes
Baking: approx. 50 minutes
Per piece: approx. 65 kcal, 5 g protein,
4 g fat, 0 g carbohydrate

Put the egg into a blender with 200 ml (¾ cup) of lukewarm water. Add the linseed, almond flour and a pinch of salt and blitz until all the ingredients have come together. Let it stand for about 10 minutes.

Line a baking tray with greaseproof paper. Spread the dough out on a baking tray using a dough scraper to create an 3–4-mm (⅛-inch) thick rectangle measuring roughly 30 × 28 cm (12 × 11 inches).

Slide the tray into the centre of the oven, then switch the oven on to 140°C (275°F) and bake the crispbread for 50 minutes.

Remove and immediately slice into ten equal-sized pieces (roughly 6 × 14 cm/2⅓ × 5½ inches). Turn off the heat, return the tray to the oven and leave the crispbread to cool completely with the door slightly ajar.

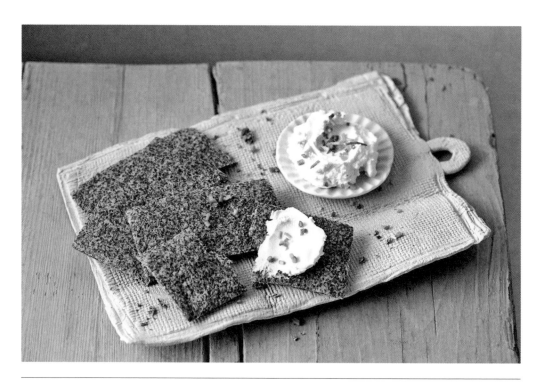

COTTAGE CHEESE FLATBREAD

250 g (8¾ oz) cottage cheese
2 medium eggs
2 tablespoons sesame seed flour
1 tablespoon ground psyllium husks
2 teaspoons black and white
   sesame seeds
salt

Makes 1
Preparation: approx. 10 minutes
Standing time: approx. 10 minutes
Baking: approx. 25 minutes
Per piece: approx. 610 kcal, 58 g protein,
33 g fat, 16 g carbohydrate

Preheat the oven to 175°C (350°F). Line a baking tray with
greaseproof paper.

Whisk together the cottage cheese, eggs and a pinch of salt.
Add the sesame seed flour and ground psyllium husks, whisk
again and let it stand for 10 minutes.

Transfer the mixture to the centre of the baking tray and use
a dough scraper to shape it into a round flatbread measuring
roughly 2 cm (¾ inch) thick and 20 cm (7 inches) in diameter.

Sprinkle with sesame seeds, slide the tray into the centre of the
oven and bake for 20–25 minutes. Remove from the oven, use
the greaseproof paper to lift the flatbread from the tray and leave
to cool completely.

ADD HERB BUTTER TO GO WITH STEAK

Topped with a classic herb butter, this bread makes a fabulous
accompaniment to grilled steak. To make this, finely chop the
leaves from 1 sprig of tarragon, 2 sprigs of thyme, 3 sprigs of
parsley and ½ bunch of chervil. Snip 1 bunch of chives into little
pieces and peel and crush 1 clove of garlic. Mix everything into
150 g (5 ounces) of soft butter and season to taste with salt and
pepper. This will keep well in the fridge for 2 weeks.

3

LUNCH

You should feel refreshed and full of energy
after your lunch. These recipes are filling and
delicious, but they won't weigh you down.
Good planning is also part of good eating
and, in turn, good health. If you are short of
time, you can prepare something the night
before, then heat it up the next day to enjoy
at your leisure.

OVEN-BAKED PRAWNS WITH TOMATOES AND BUTTON MUSHROOMS

juice of ½ lemon

1 tablespoon harissa

1 garlic clove, finely chopped or crushed

5 tablespoons coconut oil

150 g (5 oz) raw frozen king prawns
    (peeled, defrosted)

200 g (7 oz) cherry tomatoes

200 g (7 oz) button mushrooms, halved

1 small courgette, cut into 3 mm
    (⅛ in) dice

salt and pepper

Serves 2

Preparation: approx. 15 minutes

Cooking: approx. 15 minutes

Defrosting: approx. 2 hours

Per portion: approx. 335 kcal,

19 g protein, 27 g fat, 5 g C

Preheat the oven to 220°C (425°F). Line a baking tray with greaseproof paper.

Stir together the lemon juice, harissa, garlic and coconut oil. Season to taste with salt and pepper and add the prawns and vegetables. Mix everything thoroughly by hand and spread evenly over the baking tray. Bake for 12 minutes in the centre of the oven. Arrange on two plates to serve.

TRY WITH PEPPER AND AUBERGINE

Use 100 g (3½ oz) finely diced yellow pepper in place of the cherry tomatoes and ½ small aubergine instead of the courgette.

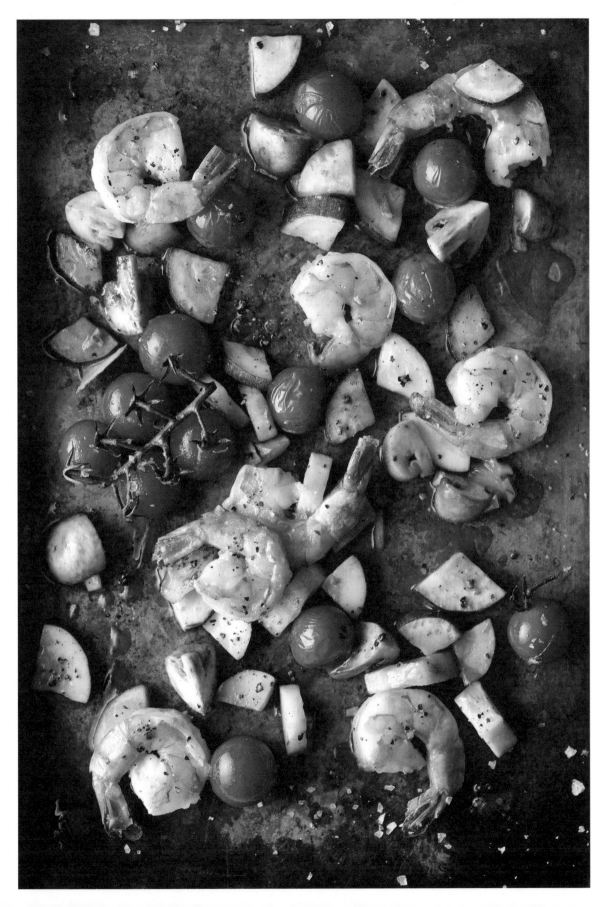

CURRY SOUP
WITH PRAWN SKEWERS

8 raw frozen king prawns (peeled,
    defrosted)
3 tablespoons coconut oil
1 carrot, peeled and finely diced
½ red pepper, deseeded and finely diced
½ leek, finely diced
2 celery stalks, finely diced
400 ml (1⅔ cups) vegetable stock
2 teaspoons curry powder
zest and juice of ½ lime
100 g (scant ½ cup) coconut milk
    (tinned)
50 g (¼ cup) cream
salt and pepper

Serves 2
Preparation: approx. 25 minutes
Defrosting: approx. 2 hours
Per portion: approx. 335 kcal,
12 g protein, 28 g fat, 7 g carbohydrate

Soak two wooden skewers for 5 minutes to prevent them from burning. Spear four prawns on each skewer.

Heat 1 tablespoon of the coconut oil in a pan over a medium heat and sauté the diced vegetables for 2 minutes. Pour over the vegetable stock and boil this down over a high heat. Add the curry powder and simmer the soup over a medium heat for about 8 minutes.

Stir the lime zest and juice, coconut milk and cream into the soup and season to taste with salt and pepper. Don't cook the soup any more, just keep it warm.

Add the remaining coconut oil to a non-stick pan over a high heat. Season the prawns with salt and pepper and sauté them for 1 minute on each side. Serve the soup in two deep bowls and garnish each with a prawn skewer.

MAKE YOUR OWN VEGETABLE BROTH

You can make your own vegetable broth by chopping up carrots, onions, potatoes and a leek. Add aromatic herbs to taste. Drop into boiling water and simmer gently for 30 minutes, then strain and discard the vegetables keeping only the liquid.

SPICY CHICKEN AND BROCCOLI SOUP

4 teaspoons clarified butter
100 g (3½ oz) broccoli, florets halved or
    quartered
50 g (1¾ oz) button mushrooms,
    quartered
2 celery stalks, diced
300 ml (1¼ cups) chicken stock
150 g (5 oz) chicken breast, chopped into
    roughly 1 cm (½ in) cubes
1 mild red chilli, finely sliced
¼ teaspoon mild paprika
½ teaspoon ground ginger
½ teaspoon ground turmeric
100 g (scant ½ cup) cream
2 tablespoons full-fat cream cheese
salt and pepper

Serves 2
Preparation: approx. 20 minutes
Per portion: approx. 435 kcal,
22 g protein, 36 g fat, 5 g carbohydrate

Heat the clarified butter in a pan over a medium heat. Add the vegetables and sauté for 2 minutes. Pour over the chicken stock, add the chicken breast and bring to the boil. Simmer, uncovered, over a medium heat for about 10 minutes.

Add the chilli, paprika, ginger and turmeric. Stir in the cream and cream cheese, and don't allow the soup to boil again. Season to taste with salt and pepper, then serve in two deep bowls.

MAKE YOUR OWN CHICKEN STOCK
You can make your own chicken broth for the week by poaching a whole chicken slowly for 90 minutes. You can add chopped leek, celery and carrot for extra flavour.

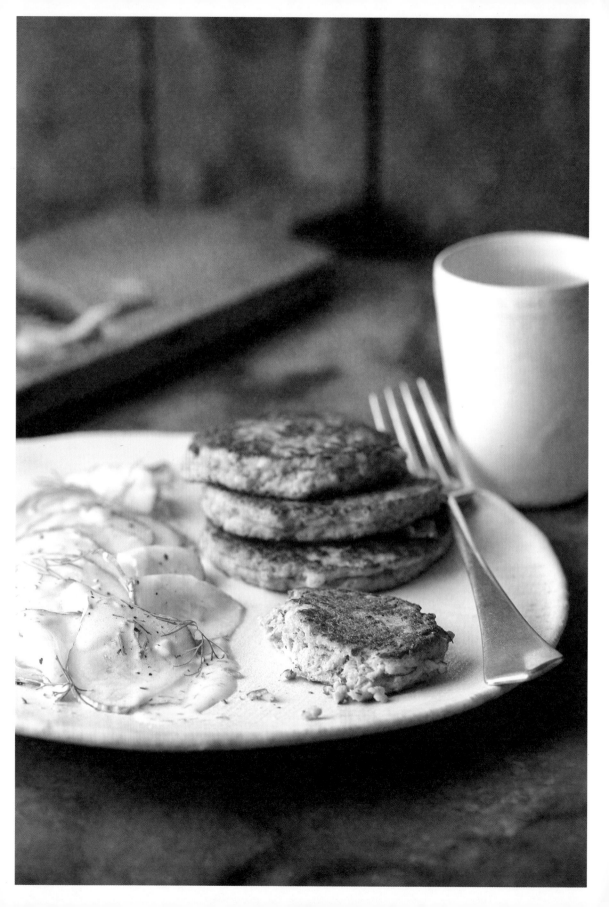

TUNA FISHCAKES WITH CUCUMBER SALAD

FOR THE FISHCAKES

1 small carrot, peeled and chopped into
    roughly 2 cm (¾ in) cubes
150-g (5-oz) tin tuna (drained weight)
2 tablespoons mayonnaise
2 medium eggs
1 tablespoon lemon juice
1 tablespoon ground psyllium husks
¼ bunch dill, finely chopped
3 teaspoons coconut oil
salt and pepper

FOR THE CUCUMBER SALAD

2 tablespoons soured cream
1 tablespoon white wine vinegar
3 teaspoons olive oil
1 teaspoon medium-hot mustard
1 cucumber, peeled and thinly sliced
salt and pepper

Serves 2
Preparation: approx. 25 minutes
Per piece: approx. 505 kcal, 27 g protein,
39 g fat, 8 g carbohydrate

Blitz the carrot, tuna, mayonnaise, eggs, lemon juice and ground psyllium husks in a food processor until finely chopped.

Fold in half the dill, reserving the rest for the cucumber salad. Season the fishcake mixture to taste with salt and pepper and let it stand for a while.

In the meantime, prepare the cucumber salad. Stir together the soured cream, white wine vinegar, olive oil and mustard. Season to taste with salt and pepper. Stir in the reserved dill. Combine all the ingredients with the sliced cucumber in a bowl and set aside.

Heat the coconut oil in a non-stick pan over a medium heat. Using moist hands, shape four flat fishcakes from the mixture and fry them for 3–4 minutes on each side. The fishcakes are fragile so use two spatulas to help you turn them.

Divide the cucumber salad between two plates, arrange the tuna fishcakes on top and serve.

FOR YOUR FREEZER

These tuna fishcakes can be frozen in batches for the perfect instant meal. Just let them defrost overnight in the fridge, then heat them up in the oven or microwave.

MARINATED TRAY-ROASTED SUMMER VEGETABLES WITH MEATBALLS

FOR THE MARINADE
juice of ½ lemon
4½ tablespoons olive oil
1 teaspoon dried basil
1 teaspoon dried oregano
salt and pepper

FOR THE VEGETABLES
1 fennel bulb, halved, stalk removed and
    thinly sliced
1 courgette, halved and cut diagonally
    into 5 mm (¼ in) slices
50 g (1¾ oz) green beans, halved
100 g (3½ oz) cherry tomatoes

FOR THE MEATBALLS
1 small onion, finely diced
20 g (¾ oz) Gouda, roughly grated
150 g (5 oz) mixed beef, pork or lamb
    mince
1 teaspoon mustard
freshly grated nutmeg
salt and pepper

Serves 2
Preparation: approx. 20 minutes
Cooking: approx. 20 minutes
Per portion: approx. 480 kcal, 22 g
protein, 40 g fat, 8 g carbohydrate

Preheat the oven to 200°C (400°F). Line a baking tray with greaseproof paper.

To make the marinade, stir the lemon juice into the olive oil, basil and oregano. Season generously to taste with salt and pepper.

Spread all the vegetables over the baking tray, mixing them together as you do so. Drizzle evenly with the marinade.

Work the onion and Gouda into the mince along with the mustard and nutmeg. Season to taste with salt and pepper. Use your hands to shape eight meatballs from the mixture, then place them on top of the vegetables and slide the tray into the centre of the oven. Bake for about 20 minutes, remove from the oven and divide between two plates to serve.

VARY YOUR VEG

There are virtually no constraints when it comes to selecting the vegetables. You can choose whatever happens to be on special offer, is in season, needs using up from your fridge or appeals to your particular tastes. It might be cauliflower, aubergine, broccoli or celery – anything goes.

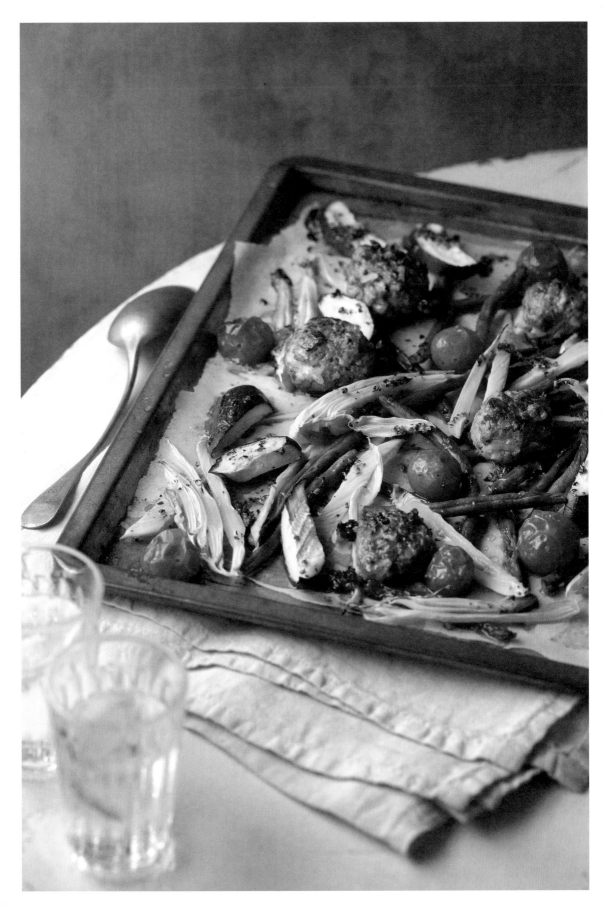

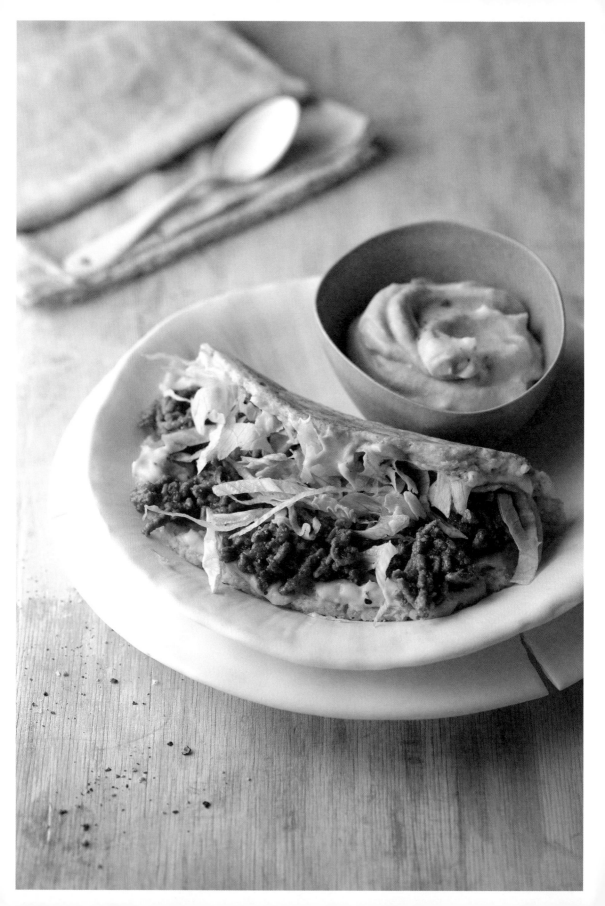

CHEESE TORTILLAS
WITH GUACAMOLE

FOR THE TORTILLAS
50 g (¾ oz) Parmesan, finely grated
2 medium eggs
100 g (⅓ cup) soured cream
50 ml (¼ cup) milk
pinch of salt
2 tablespoons ground psyllium husks
2 tablespoons sesame seed flour
2 tablespoons almond flour
1 teaspoon baking powder

FOR THE FILLING
3 teaspoons coconut oil
150 g (5 oz) beef mince
1 tablespoon tomato purée
½ teaspoon ground coriander
½ teaspoon dried oregano
100 g (3½ oz) iceberg lettuce, sliced into
   thin strips
salt and pepper

FOR THE GUACAMOLE
juice of ¼ lemon
flesh of ¼ avocado
1 tablespoon crème fraîche
salt and pepper

Serves 2
Preparation: approx. 30 minutes
Per portion: approx. 775 kcal, 48 g
protein, 59 g fat, 10 g carbohydrate

Preheat the oven to 200°C (400°F). Line a baking tray with greaseproof paper.

Stir the Parmesan together with the eggs, soured cream, milk, salt and 50 ml (¼ cup) of water in a bowl. In a second bowl, combine the ground psyllium husks, sesame seed flour, almond flour and baking powder, then swiftly stir these dry ingredients into the wet ingredients.

Divide the mixture into four and shape into balls. Arrange these on the baking tray and use damp hands to press each one flat to create a roughly 6-mm (¼-in) thick tortilla. Put the tray in the centre of the oven and bake for 10 minutes. Switch off the oven, open the door slightly and leave the tortillas inside to stay warm.

In the meantime, put the coconut oil in a pan over a medium heat and sauté the mince for about 8 minutes until crumbly and brown. Stir in the tomato purée and 1 tablespoon of water, add the coriander and oregano and season with salt and pepper.

Add the lemon juice to a blender with the avocado and crème fraîche and process until you have a purée. Season to taste with salt and pepper.

Remove the tortillas from the oven and spread evenly with the guacamole. Use a tablespoon to scoop the mince onto one half of each tortilla and then scatter the iceberg lettuce on top. Fold up the tortillas and arrange on two plates to serve.

GUACAMOLE VARIATIONS
Have you got some leftover broccoli or asparagus from a previous day? You can use these vegetables instead of avocado to make the guacamole. Just replace the avocado with 50 g (1¾ oz) cooked vegetables and create any number of fantastic alternative options.

SOUVLAKI KEBABS
WITH MARINATED FETA

FOR THE FETA

100 g (3½ oz) feta, cut into 2 cm
  (¾ in) cubes
½ red onion, thinly sliced
1 garlic clove, roughly sliced
1 mild red chilli, sliced into thin rings
1 teaspoon dried thyme
3 teaspoons olive oil
salt

FOR THE SOUVLAKI

1 tablespoon lemon juice
2 tablespoons olive oil
3 sprigs parsley, finely chopped (or
  1 tablespoon chopped frozen parsley)
½ teaspoon dried rosemary
1 teaspoon dried oregano
150 g (5 oz) pork neck, chopped into
  roughly 3 cm (1¼ in) cubes
2 yellow peppers, chopped into roughly
  3 cm (1¼ in) pieces
salt and pepper

Serves 2
Preparation: approx. 30 minutes
Marinating: approx. 1 hour
Per portion: approx. 495 kcal, 23 g
protein, 42 g fat, 5 g carbohydrate

Add all the feta ingredients to a bowl with a pinch of salt and carefully combine by hand so that the feta is nicely covered with the oil. Cover and chill in the fridge until you are ready to serve.

Mix the lemon juice with 1 tablespoon of the olive oil and the herbs in a large bowl. Season generously to taste with salt and pepper. Coat the meat with the herby marinade. Cover and chill in the fridge for 1 hour or overnight.

Meanwhile, soak two 20 cm (8 in) skewers in water for about 1 hour. Remove the meat from its marinade and alternately slide the chunks onto the skewers with two or three pieces of pepper in between.

Heat the remaining olive oil in a griddle or frying pan over medium heat. Fry the souvlaki skewers for 2–3 minutes on all sides. Any pepper pieces that didn't fit on the skewers can be fried at the same time.

Remove the garlic from the feta marinade and discard. Serve the cubed feta and marinade on two plates, arrange the souvlaki skewers on top and you are ready to eat.

LESS HEAT?

From a mild kick to infernal heat, chillies vary hugely in terms of their power. Depending on the particular variety; you may want to remove the chilli seeds and white membrane to make the heat a bit milder.

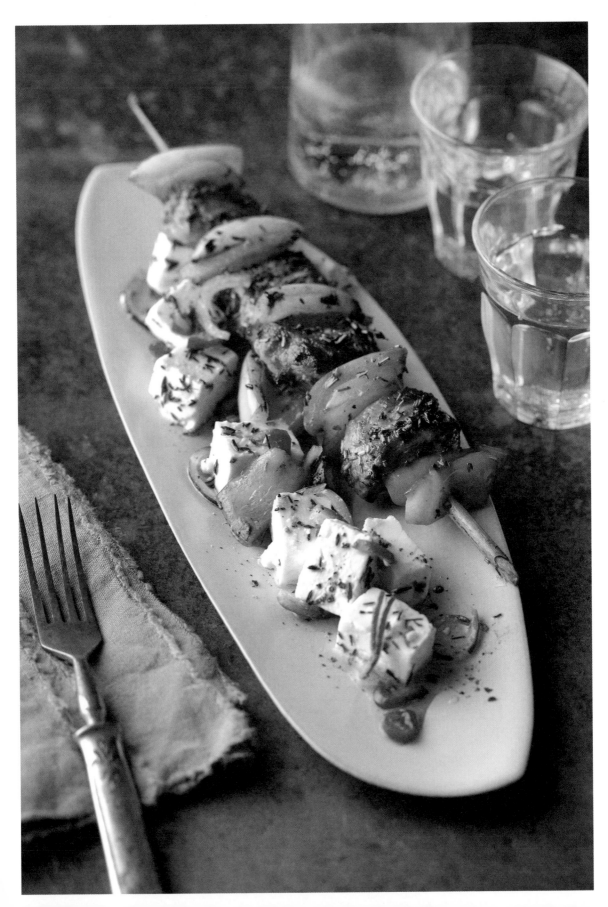

MOUSSAKA

2 aubergines, sliced lengthways into
    8-mm (⅓-in) thick slices
1 tablespoon lemon juice
3 tablespoons olive oil
100 g (3½ oz) beef mince
1 onion, finely chopped
½ teaspoon fennel seeds
200 g (7 oz) chopped tomatoes (tinned)
2½ tablespoons vegetable stock
2 bay leaves
1 teaspoon dried oregano
50 g (¾ oz) Gouda, roughly grated
1 medium egg
50 g (¼ cup) cream
freshly grated nutmeg
salt and pepper

Serves 2
Preparation: approx. 25 minutes
Cooking: approx. 45 minutes
Per portion: approx. 475 kcal, 25 g
protein, 38 g fat, 9 g carbohydrate

Preheat the oven to 220°C (425°F).

Place the aubergine slices flat on the tray. Mix the lemon juice
with 1 tablespoon of the olive oil and brush evenly over the
aubergine. Season the slices with a pinch of salt and pepper,
slide the tray into the centre of the oven and bake for 15 minutes.
Remove, then reduce the oven temperature to 180°C (350°F).

In the meantime, heat the remaining olive oil in a pan and fry the
beef mince until brown and crumbly. Add the onion and fennel
seeds. Pour over the tomatoes and stock and add the bay leaves
and oregano. Simmer everything, uncovered, for 5 minutes, then
season to taste with salt and pepper. Remove the bay leaves.

Mix the Gouda into the egg and cream. Season with a pinch salt
and some nutmeg.

Line the base of a 26 × 20 cm (10 × 8 in) baking dish with a third
of the baked aubergine slices. Spread half the mince mixture on
top. Cover with another layer of aubergine, spread the remaining
mince on top and finish with a layer of the remaining aubergine.

Pour the egg and cream sauce over the top. Transfer the baking
dish to the centre of the oven and bake the moussaka for 30
minutes. Remove from the oven and serve on two plates.

COURGETTE MOUSSAKA

You could also use 2 large courgettes instead of the aubergines.
Follow the recipe as given, but only prebake the courgette for 10
minutes, as it cooks rather more quickly than aubergine.

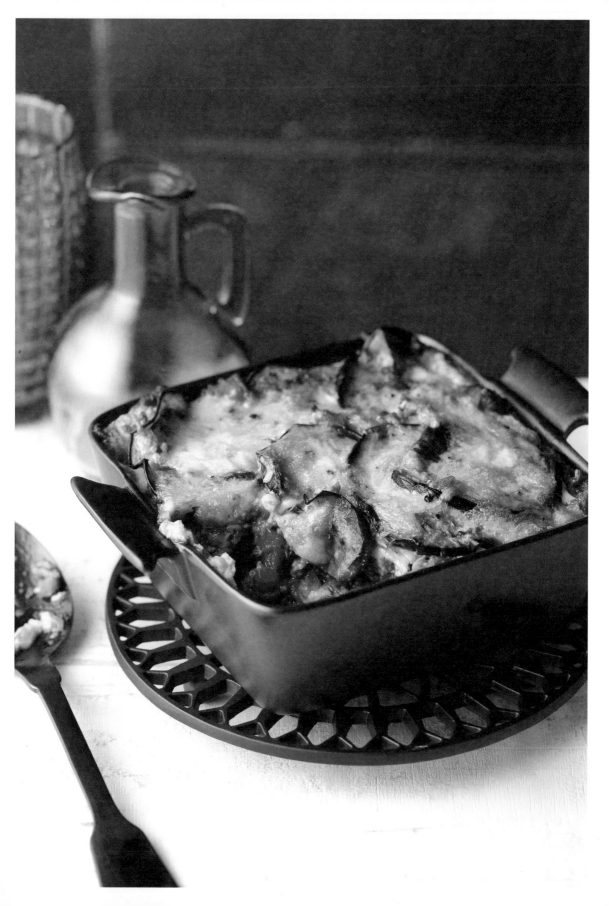

OVER-ROASTED COURGETTE

2 courgettes, quartered lengthways then
    cut into 3–4 pieces
zest of ½ lemon
1 garlic clove, finely chopped or crushed
4½ tablespoons olive oil
½ teaspoon nigella seeds
2 tablespoons sesame seeds
60 g (2 oz) Parmesan, finely grated
salt and pepper

Serves 2
Preparation: approx. 15 minutes
Cooking: approx. 20 minutes
Per portion: approx. 430 kcal, 16 g
protein, 38 g fat, 5 g carbohydrate

Preheat the oven to 200°C (400°F). Line a baking tray with greaseproof paper.

Put the courgette pieces into a bowl with the lemon zest, garlic and olive oil and toss everything by hand until the pieces are completely coated.

Spread the courgette evenly over the baking tray, season with salt and pepper and scatter over the nigella and sesame seeds. Transfer the tray to the centre of the oven and cook for 10 minutes.

Remove, sprinkle over the Parmesan, then continue baking the courgette for a further 8 minutes. Divide the roasted courgette between two plates to serve.

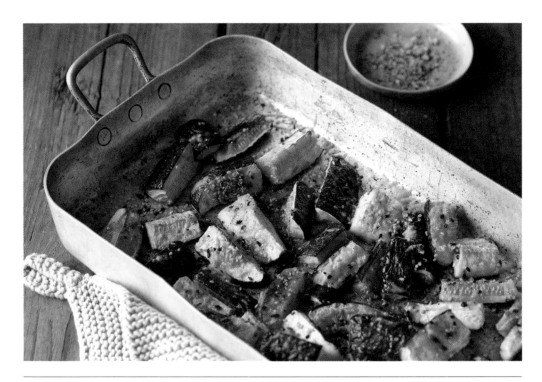

SWISS CHARD WRAPS
WITH A HAM FILLING

8 Swiss chard leaves, leaves and stalks
    separated, stalks cubed
8 slices cooked ham
4 slices Gouda, halved
8 teaspoons butter
100 ml (scant ½ cup) vegetable stock
50 g (¼ cup) cream
1 tablespoon herb cream cheese
1 teaspoon ground turmeric
salt and pepper

Serves 2
Preparation: approx. 25 minutes
Per portion: approx. 515 kcal,
37 g protein, 39 g fat, 2 g carbohydrate

Spread the Swiss chard leaves out flat on the work surface and top with the ham. Lay the Gouda slices lengthways toward the centre of the slices of ham. Fold in the sides of the Swiss chard leaves toward the centre, then roll each one up and secure with a toothpick.

Add the butter to a shallow pan over a medium heat and sauté the Swiss chard stalks for 2 minutes. Pour in the vegetable stock and cream, stir in the herb cream cheese and add the turmeric. Bring to the boil, then add the Swiss chard parcels.

Simmer the parcels, covered, for about 12 minutes over a low heat. Season the Swiss chard and cream cheese mixture with salt and pepper and then serve on two plates.

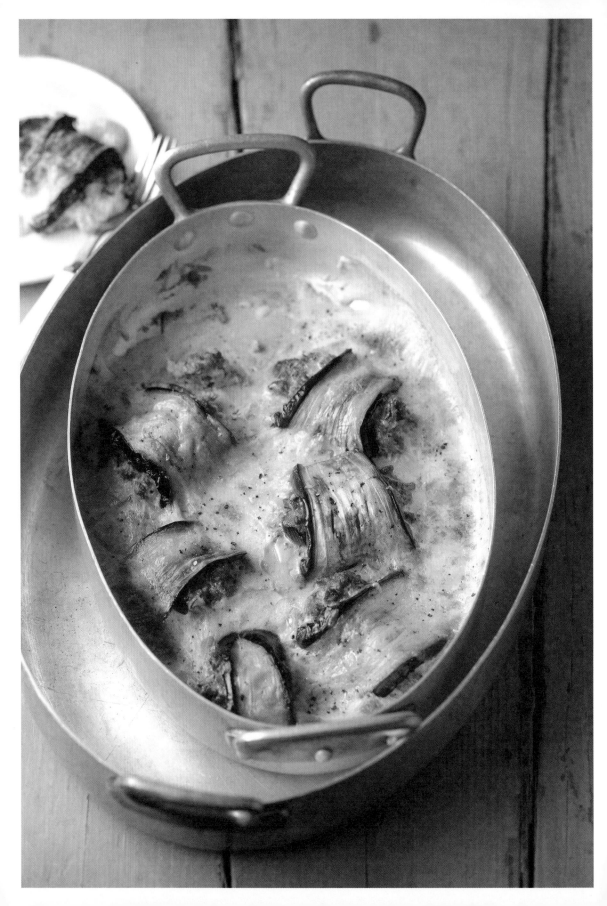

STUFFED AUBERGINE AU GRATIN

FOR THE AUBERGINE
3 teaspoons olive oil
1 aubergine, sliced lengthways into 6–8
      1-cm (½-in) thick slices
1 small red onion, finely diced
150 g (5 oz) mixed beef, pork or lamb
      mince
1 medium egg
1 teaspoon mild paprika
salt and pepper

FOR THE BÉCHAMEL SAUCE
4 teaspoons butter
1 teaspoon ground psyllium husks
pinch of ground cloves
freshly grated nutmeg
50 ml (¼ cup) milk
40 g (1½ oz) cheddar, roughly grated
salt and pepper

Serves 2
Preparation: approx. 30 minutes
Cooking: approx. 30 minutes
Per portion: approx. 500 kcal, 25 g
protein, 42 g fat, 5 g carbohydrate

Heat the olive oil in a large, non-stick pan. Sauté the sliced aubergine in the oil for 1 minute on each side, remove and drain on some kitchen paper.

Put the onion, mince and egg into a bowl and work together by hand. Add the paprika and season with salt and pepper.

Place the aubergine slices side by side on a work surface. Put 1 tablespoon of the mince mixture onto half of each aubergine slice (on the side with the largest surface area) and fold the other half over the top. Press down slightly to distribute the meat mixture. Transfer these aubergine pockets to a 26 × 20 cm (10 × 8 in) baking dish. Preheat the oven to 180°C (350°F).

Melt the butter in a pan. Using a whisk, stir the ground psyllium husks into the melted butter. Add the ground cloves, season with nutmeg, salt and pepper, then add 150 ml (⅔ cup) of water and the milk while stirring constantly. Bring to the boil over a medium heat until the sauce has thickened. This will take 2–4 minutes.

Remove the pan from the hob, stir in the cheddar and pour the sauce evenly over the aubergine parcels. Bake the dish in the centre of the oven for 25–30 minutes until the béchamel sauce is golden brown. Remove from the oven and divide between two plates to serve.

STUFFED PEPPERS
You can also use this filling for stuffed peppers. To do this, slice 1 yellow pepper in half and remove the seeds and membrane. Scoop the mince mixture into the pepper halves, then transfer them to a 20-cm (8-in) square, lightly greased baking dish. Pour over the béchamel sauce and bake as described.

COURGETTE OMELETTE
WITH SERRANO HAM

4 medium eggs
4 teaspoons cream
30 g (1 oz) pecorino, roughly grated
1 courgette, roughly grated
1 garlic clove, finely chopped or crushed
6 black olives (stoned), chopped
1 teaspoon mild paprika
3 tablespoons olive oil
1 tomato, finely diced
3 slices serrano ham
salt and pepper

Serves 2
Preparation: approx. 20 minutes
Per portion: approx. 470 kcal, 21 g
protein, 42 g fat, 4 g carbohydrate

Whisk the eggs in a bowl with the cream. Add the cheese, courgette, tomato, garlic, olives and paprika and stir well. Season with a pinch of salt and pepper.

Heat 1 tablespoon of the oil in a non-stick pan. Add the egg mixture, cover and cook over a medium heat for 8 minutes. Slip the omelette onto a plate. Place a second plate upside down over the top, then flip both plates over together to turn the omelette.

Add the remaining oil to the pan. Slide the omelette back into the pan from the second plate, cover and continue cooking for 5 minutes.

Slip the omelette onto a chopping board, slice into quarters, top with the ham and serve.

ALTERNATIVE FILLINGS

Omelettes are great for using up any leftovers. Do you have some cooked vegetables or a bit of meat that needs finishing? Chop them into little pieces and use these instead of the courgette or tomato in the egg mixture. This way you'll always be able to rustle up new varieties of omelette.

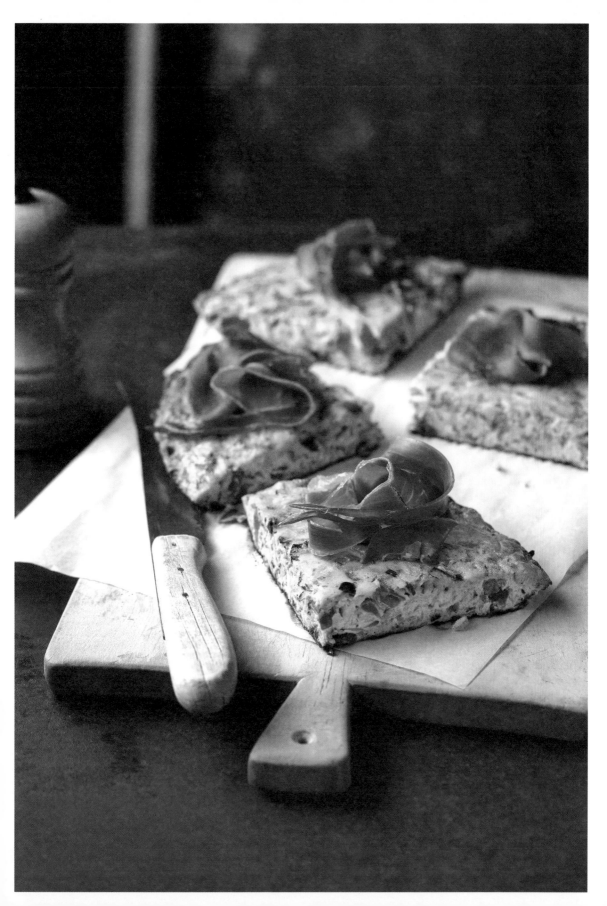

CHICKEN NUGGETS
WITH BAKED TOMATOES

2 tomatoes, halved

1½ tablespoons pine nuts, roughly
   chopped

20 g (¾ oz) Parmesan, finely grated

1 spring onion, sliced into very thin rings

1 tablespoon creamed coconut

2 tablespoons Greek yoghurt

1 teaspoon curry powder

¼ apple, finely grated

2 tablespoons ground almonds

8 teaspoons clarified butter

120 g (4½ oz) chicken breast, cut into
   roughly 3 cm (1¼ in) cubes

1 medium egg, beaten

salt and pepper

Serves 2

Preparation: approx. 35 minutes

Per portion: approx. 610 kcal,

27 g protein, 52 g fat, 8 g carbohydrate

Place the tomato halves in a 20-cm (8-in) square baking dish, cut-side up. Mix the pine nuts with the Parmesan and spring onion. Season the tomatoes with salt and pepper and sprinkle with this mixture. Slide the dish into the centre of a cold oven and set the temperature to 200°C (400°F) to cook for 25 minutes.

Meanwhile, stir together the creamed coconut, yoghurt and curry powder. Stir the apple into the curry sauce and season to taste with salt and pepper. Put the almonds on a flat plate.

Warm the clarified butter in a pan over a medium heat. Season the chicken pieces with salt and pepper and toss them in the egg, then in the almonds. Fry the pieces for 2 minutes on each side until golden brown all over. Remove from the pan, drain on kitchen paper and serve on two plates. Take the tomatoes out of the oven, arrange on the plates and serve with the curry sauce.

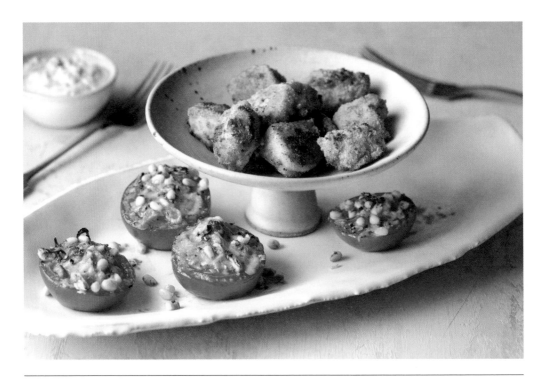

CAULIFLOWER AND TURMERIC CHEESE FRITTERS

(V)

400 g (3¼ cups) cauliflower florets
100 g (3½ oz) Gouda, roughly grated
2 medium eggs
50 g (¼ cup) full-fat cream cheese
freshly grated nutmeg
1 teaspoon ground turmeric
2 teaspoons ground psyllium husks
3 tablespoons coconut oil
salt and pepper

Serves 2
Preparation: approx. 25 minutes
Per portion: approx. 465 kcal,
29 g protein, 36 g fat, 8 g carbohydrate

Bring about 500 ml (2 cups) of water to the boil and add salt. Cook the cauliflower florets in the boiling water for 6 minutes, covered, then drain. Immerse in cold water to prevent them cooking any further, then drain again.

Meanwhile, mix the Gouda with the eggs and cream cheese.

Blitz the cauliflower in a food processor until you have fine crumbs, then add it to the egg and cheese mixture. Season with salt, pepper and nutmeg, then add the turmeric and ground psyllium husks and stir briskly. Let it stand for roughly 10 minutes.

Add the oil to a non-stick pan over a medium heat. Use damp hands to shape eight fritters from the mix and then fry for 4 minutes on each side. Remove and drain on some kitchen paper before serving.

SERVE WITH A SIDE

Mix a handful each of iceberg lettuce and radicchio cut into strips. Make a dressing by stirring together ½ teaspoon medium-hot mustard, 2 tablespoons red wine vinegar and 1 tablespoon olive oil and season generously with salt and pepper. Toss the salad in the dressing.

TOMATO AND RED PEPPER SOUP WITH PARMESAN CRISPS

(V)

FOR THE PARMESAN CRISPS
1 teaspoon chilli flakes
1 tablespoon fennel seeds
60 g (2 oz) Parmesan, finely grated

FOR THE SOUP
1 red pepper, halved and deseeded
3 tablespoons olive oil
1 small onion, finely chopped
200 g (7 oz) peeled tomatoes (tinned)
250 ml (1 cup) vegetable stock
1 teaspoon dried rosemary
2 sprigs basil, leaves picked
2 tablespoons crème fraîche
salt and pepper

Serves 2
Preparation: approx. 30 minutes
Per portion: approx. 395 kcal, 15 g
protein, 32 g fat, 10 g carbohydrate

Preheat the oven to 200°C (400°F). Line a baking tray with greaseproof paper. Crush the chilli flakes and fennel seeds using a pestle and mortar and mix with the Parmesan.

Dollop spoonfuls of the mixture on the baking tray to create six Parmesan crisps. Space them somewhat apart because they will spread. Slide the tray into the centre of the oven and bake for 4 minutes until the cheese has melted and the edges have begun to brown. Remove from the oven and leave to cool completely on a wire rack (still on the greaseproof paper). Set the oven temperature to 250°C (475°F) grill setting.

To make the soup, place the pepper pieces skin-side up on a baking tray and bake on the top shelf of the oven for 10–15 minutes until the skin begins to blister and turn black. Remove, cover with a clean, wet tea towel and leave to cool slightly.

Meanwhile, add the olive oil to a pan over a medium heat and sweat the onion for 2 minutes. Add the peeled tomatoes to the pan along with the vegetable stock, rosemary and basil and bring to the boil, uncovered. Simmer for 8–10 minutes.

Pull the skin off the pepper and add the peeled pieces to the pan. Blend with a hand blender, return to the boil and season to taste with salt and pepper.

Serve in two deep bowls, each one topped with 1 tablespoon of crème fraîche and garnished with the Parmesan crisps.

SPEED THINGS UP

This soup still tastes great without the time-consuming step of roasting the peppers to remove the skin. Once blended the skin is barely noticeable.

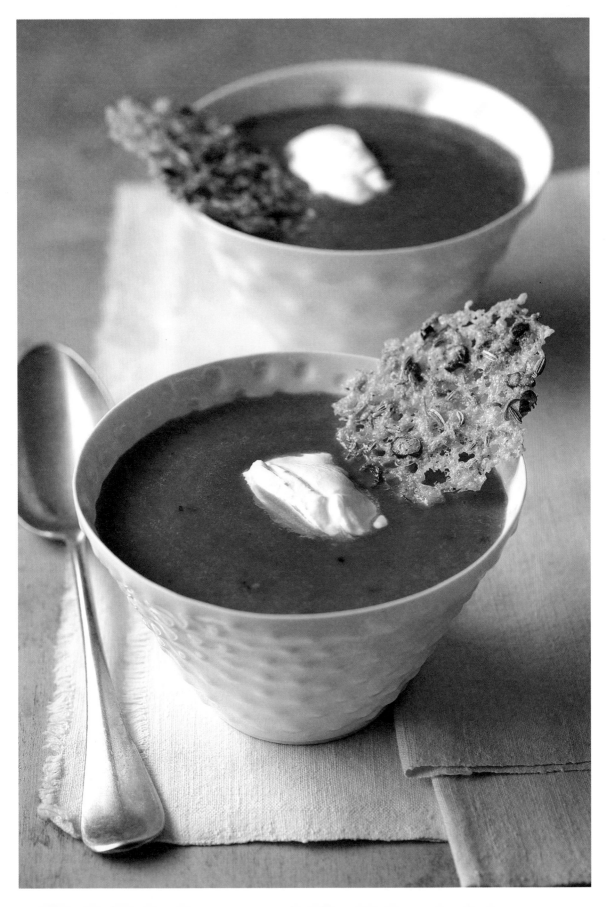

VEGGIE SPAGHETTI
WITH MUSHROOM SAUCE

(V)

FOR THE VEGGIE SPAGHETTI
1 kohlrabi, peeled and spiralized
1 large carrot, peeled and spiralized
1 small courgette, spiralized
3 sprigs parsley, roughly chopped
salt

FOR THE MUSHROOM SAUCE
8 teaspoons butter
1 small onion, finely diced
200 g (7 oz) button mushrooms, halved
    or quartered
150 g (⅔ cup) cream
50 g (¼ cup) full-fat cream cheese
½ teaspoon mild paprika
freshly grated nutmeg
salt and pepper

Serves 2
Preparation: approx. 25 minutes
Per portion: approx. 520 kcal, 10 g
protein, 48 g fat, 12 g carbohydrate

Bring approximately 6 cups (1.5 liters) of salted water to the boil in a pan. Boil the veggie spaghetti, uncovered, for 4 minutes, then drain.

Meanwhile, melt the butter in a pan over a high heat. Sauté the onion and mushrooms together for 2 minutes.

Pour in the cream, bring to the boil, uncovered, and allow to thicken slightly for 1 minute. Remove the pan from the hob and stir in the cream cheese. Add the paprika and season the mushrooms to taste with nutmeg, salt and pepper. Cover to keep warm.

Divide the veggie spaghetti between two deep plates. Pour over the mushroom sauce and scatter with chopped parsley to serve.

DELICIOUS RECYCLING

When preparing broccoli, the stalk often ends up unused in the compost, but it's ideal for making veggie spaghetti. Just peel it, then use it in exactly the same way as you would a carrot. Depending on the time of year, you can also make wonderful veggie spaghetti from sweet potato (in moderation), beetroot and pumpkin. If you don't have a spiralizer, you can use a peeler to make thin strips like tagliatelle.

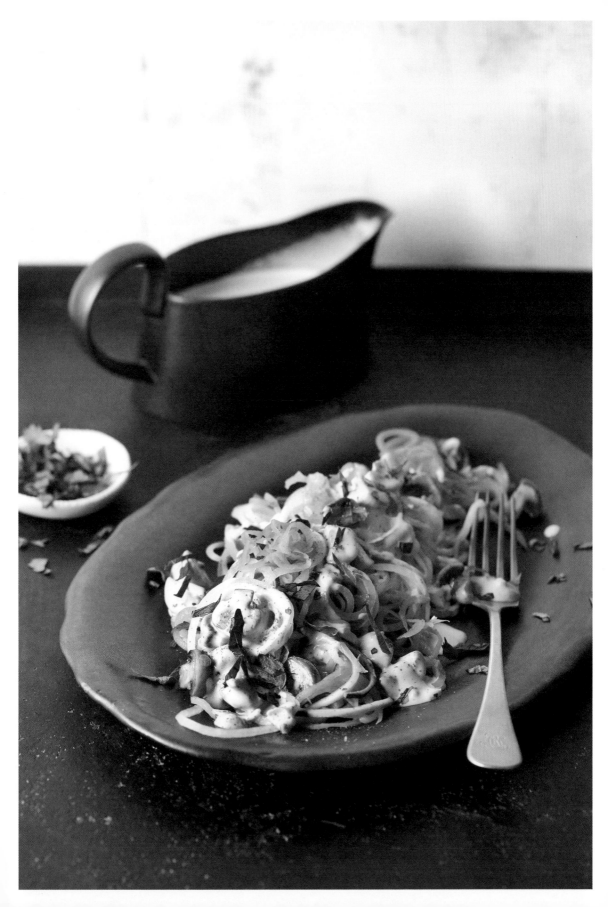

SAUERKRAUT AND BACON PATTIES

300 g (10½ oz) sauerkraut

4 rashers bacon, finely diced

1 carrot, peeled and roughly grated

50 g (1¾ oz) celeriac, peeled and roughly grated

½ red pepper, cut into thin strips

2 tablespoons ground psyllium husks

2 medium eggs

½ teaspoon nigella seeds

150 g (½ cup) Greek yoghurt

1 tablespoon ajvar

3 tablespoons coconut oil

salt and pepper

Serves 2

Preparation: approx. 25 minutes

Per portion: approx. 340 kcal,

9 g protein, 29 g fat, 10 g carbohydrate

Fork through the sauerkraut and add the bacon and vegetables. Add the ground psyllium husks, eggs, nigella seeds and a pinch each of salt and pepper. Combine the mixture with your hands and let it stand for 10 minutes.

Stir together the yoghurt and ajvar and season to taste with salt and pepper. Melt the coconut oil in a non-stick pan over a low heat. With damp hands, shape six flat patties from the mixture and then fry them in the covered pan for 5–6 minutes on each side. Arrange the patties on two plates and serve with the dip.

PUMPKIN AND SAUERKRAUT PATTIES

Replace the carrot, celeriac and pepper with 200 g (7 oz) pumpkin (Hokkaido or butternut squash). Roughly grate the pumpkin or squash, then proceed as described above.

CAULIFLOWER AND SPINACH BAKE

1 small cauliflower, split into florets
8 teaspoons butter
1 small onion, finely diced
200 g (7 oz) spinach
50 g (¼ cup) cream
125 g (4½ oz) ball mozzarella, diced or
    grated
50 g (1¾ oz) Gouda, roughly grated
pinch of ground cloves
freshly grated nutmeg
salt and pepper

Serves 2
Preparation: approx. 25 minutes
Cooking: approx. 20 minutes
Per portion: approx. 495 kcal, 25 g
protein, 41 g fat, 6 g carbohydrate

In a medium pan, bring roughly 6 cups (1.5 liters) of water to the boil and add salt. Boil the cauliflower florets for 8 minutes until just done, then briefly drain.

Meanwhile, heat 4 teaspoons of the butter in a shallow pan. Sauté the onion for 1 minute, then add the spinach and let it wilt before setting the pan aside. Preheat the oven to 200°C (400°F).

Blitz the cauliflower in a food processor with the cream and the remaining butter until crumbly. Mix with the spinach, mozzarella and Gouda. Add the cloves and season with nutmeg, salt and pepper. Transfer to a 20-cm (8-in) square baking dish and cook in the centre of the oven for 20 minutes until the cheese is golden brown. Remove from the dish and serve on two plates.

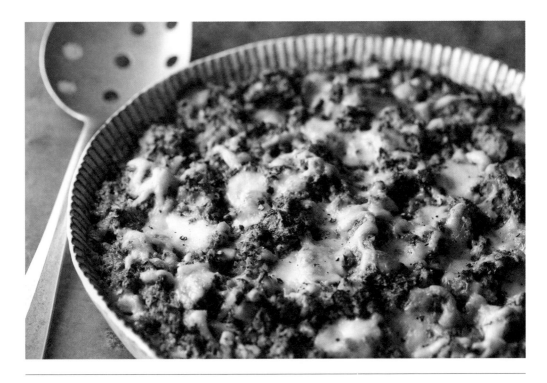

BRAISED PORK TENDERLOIN
WITH PAPRIKA MUSHROOMS

200 g (7 oz) pork tenderloin, sliced into
    roughly 4 cm (1½ in) cubes
3 tablespoons coconut oil
1 small onion, thinly sliced
1 tablespoon tomato purée
400 ml (1¾ cups) meat stock
4 teaspoons butter
400 g (14 oz) button mushrooms,
    quartered
100 g (scant ½ cup) cream
½ teaspoon dried thyme
1 teaspoon mild paprika
freshly grated nutmeg
salt and pepper

Serves 2
Preparation: approx. 45 minutes
Per portion: approx. 515 kcal, 29 g
protein, 43 g fat, 5 g carbohydrate

Generously season the pork tenderloin with salt and pepper. Put
the coconut oil in a pan over a medium heat and sauté the meat
on all sides for 5 minutes until golden brown.

Add the onion to the pan and continue frying for 10 minutes.
Once the meat and onion have acquired plenty of colour, stir
in the tomato purée and cook for a further 1 minute.

Pour over the stock and cover the pan with a lid. Braise for
30 minutes over a medium heat. Check occasionally to make
sure there is enough liquid in the pan and top up with hot water
if necessary.

Meanwhile, melt the butter in a pan over a medium heat and
sauté the mushrooms briskly until they begin to brown. Add
the mushrooms to the meat and pour in the cream.

Bring to the boil over a high heat and simmer for 4–5 minutes to
reduce the sauce to a creamy consistency. Add the dried thyme
and paprika and season with some nutmeg, salt and pepper.
Serve on two plates.

A TASTY ALTERNATIVE
Braising means the pork tenderloin won't get too dry. If
preferred, you can use diced pork neck instead. The stewing
meat will need about 20 minutes longer to cook to make sure
it is nice and soft once braised. You will need to keep checking
the liquid levels and topping the dish up with hot water. Most
of the liquid will be cooked off subsequently when you reduce
the sauce.

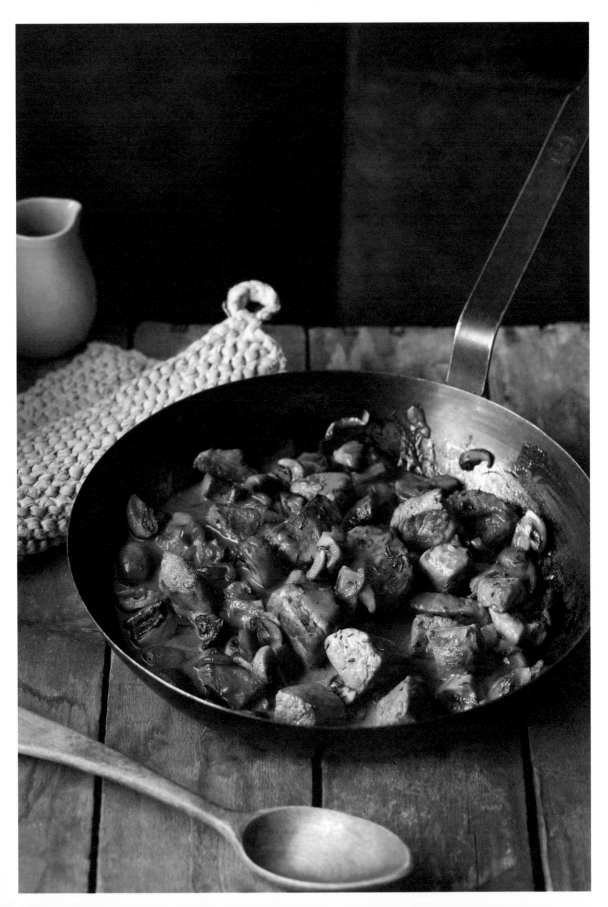

COUNTRY CASSEROLE
WITH YELLOW PEPPER

3 tablespoons coconut oil

200 g (7 oz) beef mince

1 small red onion, finely diced

1 tablespoon tomato purée

150 g (5 oz) button mushrooms,
    quartered

1 small courgette, cubed

1 yellow pepper, diced into 2 cm (¾ in)
    cubes

1 mild red chilli, sliced into thin rings

450 ml (scant 2 cups) vegetable stock

2 bay leaves

1 teaspoon dried thyme

2 tablespoons full-fat cream cheese

salt and pepper

Serves 2

Preparation: approx. 25 minutes

Per portion: approx. 450 kcal, 26 g
protein, 35 g fat, 7 g carbohydrate

Put the oil in a pan over a medium heat. Fry the mince until browned, stirring frequently. Add the onion to the pan and continue cooking.

Stir the tomato purée into the mince and cook for 1 minute. Add the vegetables and chilli and pour over the vegetable stock. Add the bay leaves and thyme and bring to the boil. Reduce to a medium heat and simmer, uncovered, for 8–10 minutes. Stir in the cream cheese, season with salt and pepper and serve immediately.

A HINT OF SPICE

Prepare this dish with lamb mince and flavour with ½ teaspoon each of ground cumin and coriander, 1 teaspoon of ras el hanout (or other chilli mix) and 6 mint leaves cut into strips.

COURGETTE AND MOZZARELLA
BOATS WITH A HERB SAUCE

2 small courgette, halved lengthways

120 g (4½ oz) mixed beef, pork or lamb mince

125 g (4½ oz) ball mozzarella, finely diced

1 teaspoon dried rosemary

4 rashers bacon

50 g (¼ cup) cream

2 tablespoons herb cream cheese

salt and pepper

Serves 2

Preparation: approx. 20 minutes

Cooking: approx. 25 minutes

Per portion: approx. 525 kcal, 31 g protein, 42 g fat, 5 g carbohydrate

Preheat the oven to 200°C (400°F). Use a spoon to hollow out the courgette slightly, then chop up the scooped-out flesh and add it to a bowl with the mince.

Add the mozzarella to the mince and work everything together using your hands until well combined. Add rosemary, salt and pepper and transfer into the courgette halves. Top each courgette boat with a rasher of bacon. Transfer them to a 26 × 20 cm (10 × 8 in) baking dish and then into the centre of the oven and bake for 15 minutes.

Stir together the cream, herb cream cheese and 1 tablespoon of water until smooth. Briefly take the dish out of the oven, pour the herby cream sauce over the courgette and return the dish to the oven. Cook for a further 10 minutes. Remove and serve the courgette on two plates.

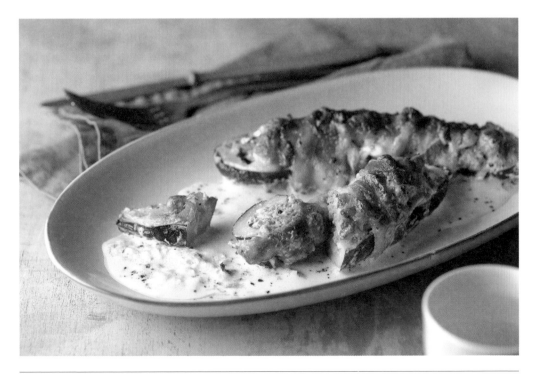

BEEF SOUP

250 g (9 oz) beef for stewing (shank or
    brisket)
bunch of soup vegetables (carrot,
    celeriac, leek)
1 onion
1 garlic clove
4 juniper berries
½ teaspoon dried thyme
½ teaspoon black peppercorns
8 teaspoons butter
3 sprigs parsley, finely chopped
salt

Serves 2
Preparation: approx. 20 minutes
Cooking: approx. 2 hours
Per portion: approx. 510 kcal, 24 g
protein, 44 g fat, 5 g carbohydrate

Add the stewing meat to a pan and cover with 6 cups (1.5 liters)
of cold water. Bring to the boil, uncovered, over a medium heat,
then lower the temperature so that it just simmers gently.

Meanwhile, prepare the soup vegetables. Wash and peel the
carrot and celeriac, carefully clean the leek. Add any peelings
into the pan with the meat. Set aside the soup vegetables.

Halve the unpeeled onion, fry it in a dry non-stick pan, cut-
surface facing down until it is almost black, then add it with
skin still on to the meat pan. Crush the unpeeled garlic clove
and add this to the pan. Grind the juniper berries using a pestle
and mortar and add these to the pan along with the thyme and
peppercorns.

Simmer the broth, uncovered, for 2 hours. If necessary, lower
the temperature to prevent it boiling too vigorously. If any foam
appears on the surface you should scoop this off using a slotted
spoon. After the 2 hours, remove the meat from the stock and
leave to cool slightly.

Meanwhile, chop the prepared soup vegetables into roughly
1 cm (½ in) cubes. Heat the butter in a large pan and sauté the
chopped vegetables for 5 minutes. Pour the stock through a fine
sieve directly onto the vegetables in the pan and bring to the
boil. Simmer for 10 minutes.

Meanwhile, chop the meat into 1 cm (½ in) cubes and add these
to the soup. Season the soup with salt, scatter over the parsley
and serve in two soup bowls.

STOCK ON SUPPLY

Making a rich stock using beef involves a bit of work and takes
some time – but it's well worth the effort for the flavour. To make
it even more worthwhile, why not prepare four times the quantity
of stock then decant it into three or four sterile jam jars while
still boiling hot. If stored in the fridge, these will keep for up to
3 months.

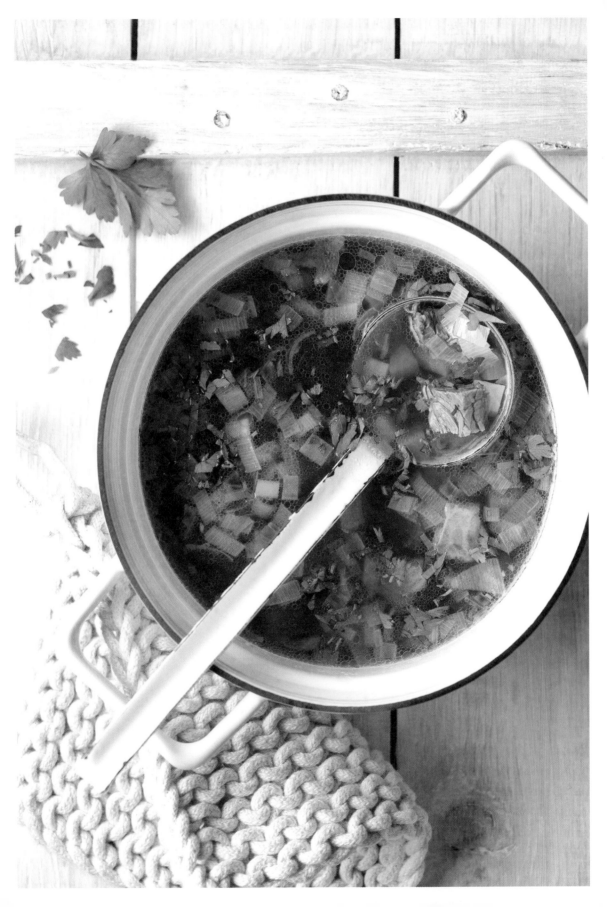

4

DINNER

Whether slow bakes or fast schnitzel, dinner needs
to be something worth coming home for. Think
ahead and be sure you have everything organized
before you get started in the kitchen. Take your
time. Good things are worth waiting for.

PORK MEDALLIONS WITH
A TOMATO AND PEPPER MEDLEY

FOR THE BASIL BUTTER
70 g (2½ oz) soft butter
zest of ¼ lemon
6 basil leaves, sliced into thin strips
salt and pepper

FOR THE MEDALLIONS
AND VEGETABLES
3 teaspoons coconut oil
200 g (7 oz) pork tenderloin, sliced into
    4 medallions
3 teaspoons olive oil
1 red onion, thinly sliced
2 yellow peppers, diced into
    2 cm (¾ in) cubes
100 g (3½ oz) cherry tomatoes, halved
4 sage leaves, sliced into thin strips
1 garlic clove, finely chopped or crushed
salt and pepper

Serves 2
Preparation: approx. 25 minutes
Per portion: approx. 550 kcal, 25 g
protein, 47 g fat, 8 g carbohydrate

To make the basil butter, beat the butter in a bowl until smooth. Stir in the lemon zest and the strips of basil. Season to taste with salt and pepper and chill until ready to serve.

Heat the coconut oil in a heavy-based pan. Season the medallions with salt and pepper and fry them on each side for 3–4 minutes.

Meanwhile, heat the olive oil in another pan and sauté the onion for 1 minute. Add the peppers and continue cooking for 2 minutes. Add the cherry tomatoes, sage and garlic, season generously with salt and pepper and mix well. Cook for another 2 minutes. Put two pork medallions on each plate and serve with the vegetables and basil butter.

HERB BUTTER VARIATIONS

Other herbs in the herb butter also work well with the medallions. For instance, you could replace the basil with 1 tablespoon of chives snipped into little pieces or 2–3 wild garlic leaves cut into thin strips. You could also use the finely chopped leaves from a sprig of rosemary or the little leaves from 2–4 sprigs of thyme.

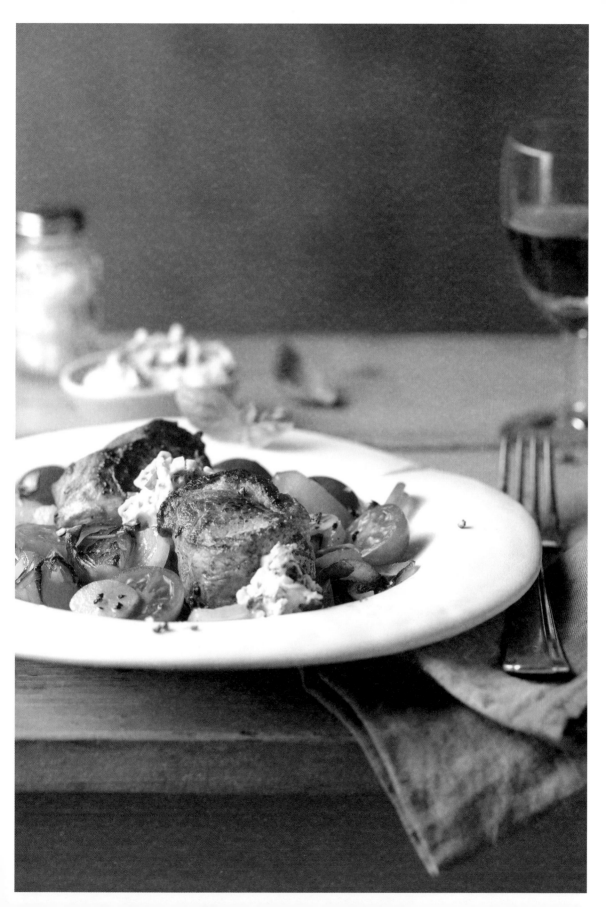

COURGETTE LASAGNA
WITH SOY BOLOGNESE

(V)

150 ml (⅔ cup) vegetable stock
50 g (⅓ cup/1¾ oz) fine textured
    soy protein
4½ tablespoons olive oil
2 small courgettes, sliced lengthways
    into 5 slices each
1 small onion, finely diced
150 g (5 oz) passata
1 teaspoon dried basil
1 teaspoon dried thyme
salt and pepper

FOR THE BÉCHAMEL SAUCE
4 teaspoons butter
½ teaspoon ground psyllium husks
freshly grated nutmeg
pinch of ground cloves
50 g (¼ cup) cream
20 g (¾ oz) Parmesan, finely grated
salt and pepper

Serves 2
Preparation: approx. 30 minutes
Cooking: approx. 25 minutes
Per portion: approx. 510 kcal, 19 g
protein, 43 g fat, 11 g carbohydrate

Bring the vegetable stock to the boil, stir in the textured soy protein, remove the pan from the heat and leave the soy granules to stand for roughly 15 minutes.

Put 2 tablespoons of the olive oil in a pan over a medium heat and sauté the courgette slices for 1 minute on each side, then remove from the pan. Put the remaining oil in a pan over a medium heat and sauté the onion for 2 minutes until it begins to take on a bit of colour. Pour in the passata, add the soaked textured soy protein and bring everything to the boil. Cover and simmer over a low heat for 10 minutes, add the basil and thyme, then season to taste with salt and pepper.

Put half the sauce into a 20-cm (8-in) square baking dish and place five slices of courgette on top, arranging them side by side. Cover with the remaining sauce, followed by the remaining courgette slices. Preheat the oven to 200°C (400°F).

For the béchamel sauce, melt the butter in a shallow pan over a medium heat. Stir the ground psyllium husks into the melted butter with a whisk. Add a pinch of nutmeg and the ground cloves, season with salt and pepper and pour in 50 ml (¼ cup) water and the cream, stirring continuously. Simmer over a medium heat until the sauce thickens. Remove the pan from the heat, stir in the Parmesan and pour the sauce evenly over the courgette lasagna.

Bake in the centre of the oven for 20–25 minutes until the béchamel sauce is golden brown. Serve on two plates.

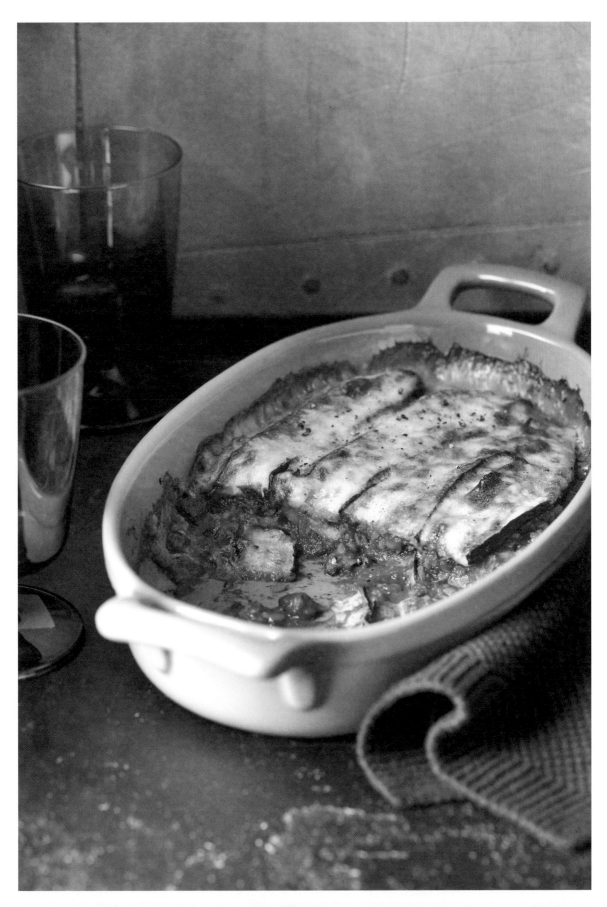

MEATBALLS WITH ASPARAGUS SALAD

3 teaspoons olive oil

400 g (14 oz) green asparagus, sliced
    into 3 cm (1¼ in) pieces

80 ml (⅓ cup) vegetable stock

¾ bunch radishes, quartered

sprig of tarragon, leaves finely chopped

1 tablespoon white wine vinegar

1 small red onion, finely chopped

1 garlic clove, finely chopped

250 g (9 oz) mince (beef and pork)

1 medium egg

1 tablespoon mustard

1 tablespoon coconut flour

freshly grated nutmeg

3 teaspoons coconut oil

salt and pepper

Serves 2
Preparation: approx. 30 minutes
Per portion: approx. 580 kcal, 36 g
protein, 45 g fat, 8 g carbohydrate

Put the olive oil in a large pan over a medium heat. Sauté the asparagus pieces for 2 minutes, pour in the vegetable stock and simmer over a medium heat for 10 minutes.

In a bowl, toss the radishes and tarragon leaves with the asparagus and vinegar. Season to taste with salt and pepper and let it stand.

In the meantime, prepare the meatballs. Add the onion and garlic to a bowl with the mince, egg, mustard and coconut flour and combine. Season to taste with nutmeg, salt and pepper.

Use your hands to form 12 equal-size balls from the mixture. Heat the coconut oil in a non-stick pan and fry the meatballs for 3–4 minutes on all sides. Divide the salad between two plates and arrange the meatballs on top to serve.

CHICKEN IN BUTTERMILK SAUCE

100 ml (scant ½ cup) buttermilk
3 tablespoons olive oil
1 teaspoon mild ground paprika
4 chicken drumsticks
8 teaspoons butter
300 g (10½ oz) white asparagus, peeled
    and woody ends trimmed
100 ml (scant ½ cup) vegetable stock
juice of ½ lemon
4 sprigs flat-leaf parsley, finely chopped,
    plus leaves to serve
salt and pepper

Serves 2
Preparation: approx. 25 minutes
Cooking: approx. 40 minutes
Per portion: approx. 465 kcal, 18 g
protein, 41 g fat, 5 g carbohydrate

Preheat the oven to 200°C (400°F). Make a marinade from the buttermilk, olive oil and ground paprika and season generously. Lay the chicken drumsticks in a 26 × 20 cm (10 × 8 in) baking dish. Pour over the marinade and bake for 40 minutes.

Meanwhile, melt the butter in a pan over a medium heat and sauté the asparagus on all sides for a few minutes until it has begun to take on a bit of colour. Pour in the vegetable stock and season with a pinch of salt. Add the lemon juice, cover and simmer the asparagus for 15–18 minutes over a low heat.

Serve the asparagus on two plates and arrange the chicken drumsticks on top. Put the buttermilk juices into a blender along with the liquid from the asparagus and process. Stir in the parsley and season to taste with salt and pepper. Garnish the chicken drumsticks and asparagus with the reserved parsley leaves and serve with the sauce.

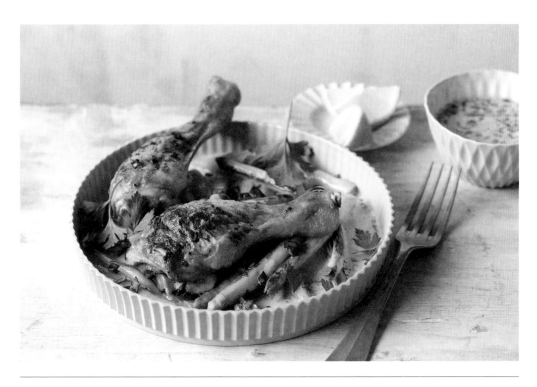

STUFFED SCHNITZEL
WITH AN ALMOND CRUST

FOR THE VEGETABLES

2 teaspoons clarified butter

1 carrot, peeled and sliced into 3 mm
(⅛ in) discs

1 courgette, sliced into 5 mm (¼ in) discs

100 g (⅔ cup) cherry tomatoes

50 ml (¼ cup) vegetable stock

salt and pepper

FOR THE SCHNITZEL

1 medium egg, beaten

25 g (¼ cup) ground almonds

1 pork schnitzel (approx. 150 g/5 oz),
halved

40 g (1½ oz) Gorgonzola, chopped

6 teaspoons clarified butter

salt and pepper

Serves 2

Preparation: approx. 25 minutes

Per portion: approx. 505 kcal, 28 g
protein, 40 g fat, 6 g carbohydrate

To make the schnitzel, put the beaten egg into a deep dish and tip the ground almonds onto a flat plate. Place the schnitzel halves alongside each other in a freezer bag and bash them with a meat tenderizer until they are roughly 3 mm (⅛ in) thick. Scatter the Gorgonzola pieces over the schnitzels. Fold the schnitzels over and season with salt and pepper. Toss first in the beaten egg and then in the almonds.

To make the vegetables, heat the clarified butter in a pan over a medium heat. First sauté the carrots for 2 minutes, then add the courgette and cherry tomatoes and continue cooking for a further 1 minute. Pour the stock over the vegetables and cook over a medium heat for 5 minutes.

Meanwhile, to cook the schnitzel, add the clarified butter to a non-stick pan over a medium heat. Fry the coated schnitzel for 4 minutes on each side. Remove the pan with the vegetables from the hob and leave it to one side until the schnitzel are ready.

Remove the schnitzel from the pan and leave to drain on some kitchen paper. Season the vegetables with salt and pepper and arrange on two plates. Place the schnitzel alongside the vegetables and serve.

CHOICE OF CHEESE

Of course, you can replace the Gorgonzola with any other kind of blue cheese; this only makes a very small difference in terms of the taste. If you are not so keen on the strong flavour of Gorgonzola, just substitute a milder cheese such as mozzarella, Camembert or Gouda.

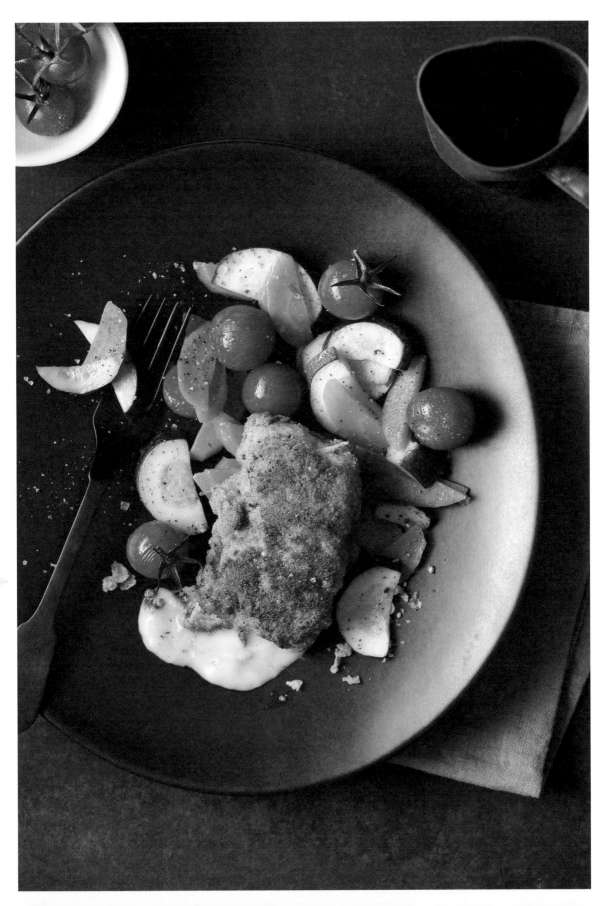

CHICKEN CURRY WITH STUFFED MUSHROOMS

FOR THE MUSHROOMS

100 g (¾ cup) frozen cauliflower florets
1 teaspoon butter, plus extra for greasing
160 g (1½ cup) brown mushrooms, stalks
    removed
50 g (¼ cup) cream
freshly grated nutmeg
20 g (¾ oz) Parmesan, finely grated
salt and pepper

FOR THE CHICKEN BREAST

4 teaspoons clarified butter
150 g (5 oz) chicken breast, sliced into
    1 cm (½ in) strips
1 small onion, finely sliced
50 g (scant ¼ cup) coconut milk (tinned)
1 tablespoon creamed coconut
1 teaspoon curry powder
salt and pepper

Serves 2
Preparation: approx. 30 minutes
Per portion: approx. 455 kcal, 25 g
protein, 37 g fat, 4 g carbohydrate

In a small pan, bring 500 ml (2 cups) water to the boil and add salt. Boil the frozen cauliflower florets for 10 minutes, then drain.

Preheat the oven to 180°C (350°F). Grease the base of a 20-cm (8-in) square baking dish with butter. Place the mushrooms, open side up in the baking dish.

Put the cream and butter into the pan used to cook the cauliflower and bring to the boil, adding a pinch of freshly grated nutmeg. Add the cauliflower and process with a hand blender until it is smooth. Stir in the Parmesan and season the mix to taste with salt and pepper.

Scoop the cauliflower purée into the upturned mushrooms. Slide the dish into the centre of the oven and cook the mushrooms for 15 minutes.

Add the clarified butter to a pan over a medium heat. Season the chicken strips with salt and pepper and fry on all sides for 3 minutes. Add the sliced onion and continue cooking for 2 minutes. Pour in the coconut milk, then stir in the creamed coconut and curry powder. Bring to the boil and season to taste with salt and pepper.

Arrange the chicken breast with the curry sauce on two plates. Remove the mushrooms from the oven, add them to the plates and serve.

PORK CHOPS WITH AVOCADO
AND APPLE SALAD

FOR THE SALAD

½ tart apple (e.g. Granny Smith), cored,
    quartered and sliced very thin
½ avocado, peeled, destoned and
    chopped into 1 cm (½ in) cubes
juice of ½ lemon
1 teaspoon mustard
3 teaspoons olive oil
½ teaspoon ground coriander
1 mild red chilli, deseeded and
    finely chopped
¼ iceberg lettuce, sliced into roughly
    1 cm (½ in) strips
salt

FOR THE PORK CHOPS

3 teaspoons coconut oil
2 pork chops (approx. 100 g/3½ oz each)
60 g (generous ¼ cup) cream
1 teaspoon green peppercorns in brine
salt and pepper

Serves 2
Preparation: approx. 20 minutes
Per portion: approx. 525 kcal, 23 g
protein, 44 g fat, 5 g carbohydrate

Add the apple to a bowl with the avocado and drizzle over
the lemon juice.

Put the coconut oil in a pan over a high heat. Season the pork
chops on both sides with salt and pepper. Fry the chops for
2 minutes on each side.

Meanwhile, make a dressing for the salad by stirring together the
mustard, olive oil, coriander and chilli. Toss the avocado, apple
and iceberg lettuce in the dressing. Season to taste with salt.

Remove the pork chops from the pan and wrap in foil to keep
warm. Deglaze the pan with the cream, then add the green
peppercorns with 1 teaspoon of the brine and simmer until the
cream sauce has thickened. Season to taste with salt and pepper.

Arrange the pork chops on two plates and drizzle over the sauce.
Serve the salad alongside.

LEAVE OUT THE GREEN PEPPERCORNS

Don't like green peppercorns? The sauce still tastes
delicious without them. It's also particularly tasty if you add
½ teaspoon mild ground paprika or the finely chopped leaves
from a sprig of rosemary.

LAMB FILLET WITH A PARSLEY AND MUSTARD TOPPING

**FOR THE COURGETTE
AND BEAN PARCELS**
4 rashers bacon
1 courgette, halved crossways and each
    half cut lengthways into four strips
50 g (1¾ oz) green beans, trimmed
8 teaspoons clarified butter

FOR THE LAMB FILLETS
3 sprigs of parsley, finely chopped
10 g (⅓ oz) Parmesan, finely grated
2 tablespoons ground almonds
2 lamb fillets (saddle of lamb, bone
    removed, each approx. 100 g/3½ oz)
3 teaspoons olive oil
1 teaspoon English mustard
salt and pepper

Serves 2
Preparation: approx. 25 minutes
Per portion: approx. 550 kcal, 30 g
protein, 46 g fat, 4 g carbohydrate

Preheat the oven to 200°C (400°F). Line a baking tray with greaseproof paper.

Spread the bacon on a work surface. Place two courgette strips and a quarter of the beans on the end of each strip, then roll up the bacon.

Mix the parsley and Parmesan with the ground almonds.

Season the lamb fillets with salt and pepper. Add the olive oil to a pan over a medium heat. Fry the lamb fillets for 2 minutes on each side. Remove from the pan and lay them on the baking tray.

Brush the top of each fillet with mustard. Spread the almond and parsley mixture evenly on top in a thick layer. Slide the tray into the centre of the oven and bake the lamb fillets for 10 minutes.

Meanwhile, heat the clarified butter in the same pan in which you fried the lamb and sauté the courgette and bean parcels for 2 minutes on each side. Add 3 tablespoons of water, reduce to a low heat, cover and continue cooking for 10 minutes.

Place two courgette bean parcels on each plate. Remove the lamb from the oven and slice each fillet twice diagonally on a chopping board to serve.

TRY RATATOUILLE WITH LAMB
Finely dice 1 small onion and sauté in 1 tablespoon of olive oil. Add 100 g (3½ oz) each of cubed aubergine, yellow pepper and courgette and sauté for 1 minute along with the onion. Add 200 g (7 oz) chopped tomatoes (tinned), cover and simmer over a low heat for 15 minutes. Add ½ teaspoon each of dried basil and oregano and season with some salt and pepper.

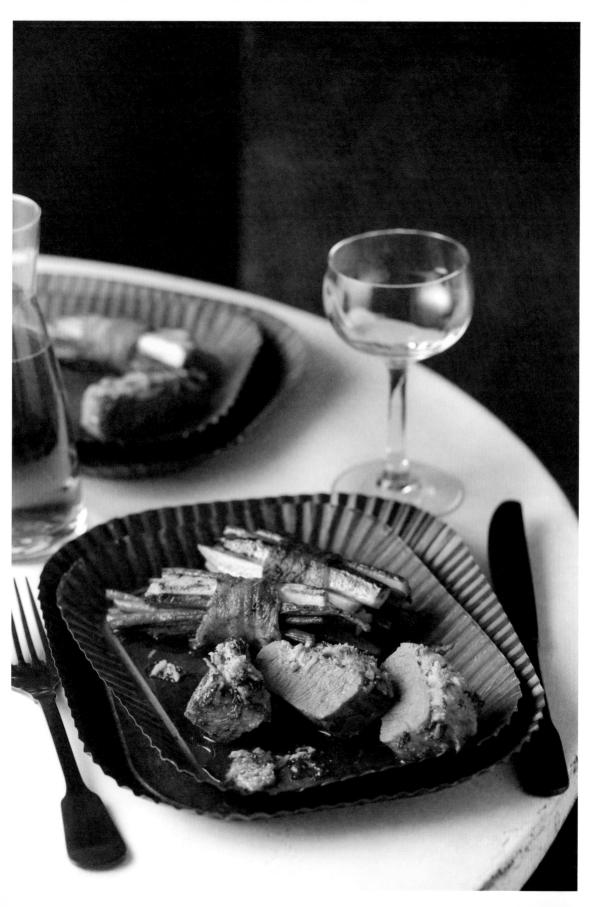

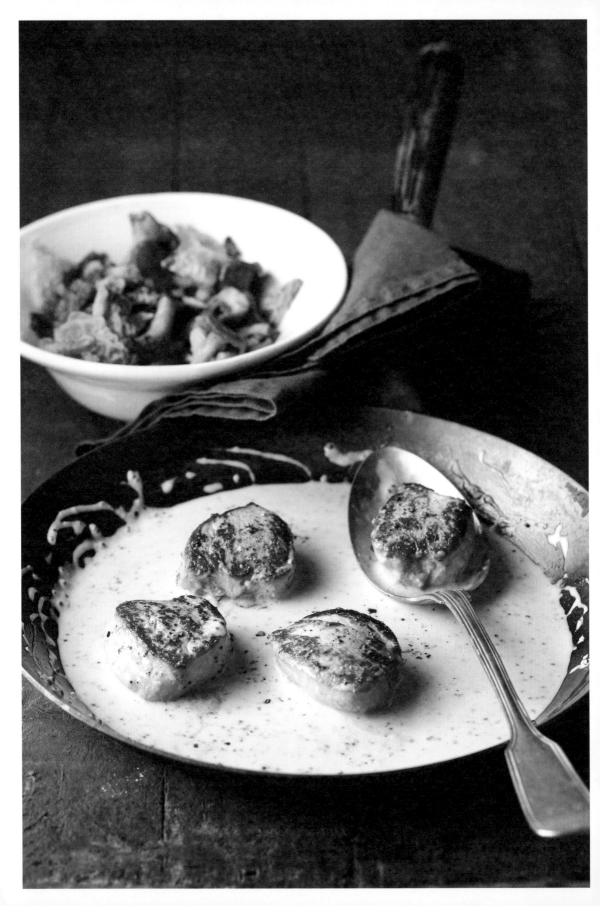

PORK TENDERLOIN IN MUSTARD SAUCE WITH SAVOY CABBAGE AND MUSHROOMS

FOR THE VEGETABLES

4 teaspoons clarified butter

200 g (7 oz) Savoy cabbage, stalk removed and leaves thinly sliced

5 rashers bacon, diced or sliced into strips

100 g (3½ oz) small button mushrooms, or mixed wild mushrooms if you have them (e.g. chanterelles, bay bolete mushrooms, porcini), halved or quartered depending on size

100 ml (scant ½ cup) vegetable stock

freshly grated nutmeg

salt and pepper

FOR THE PORK TENDERLOIN

3 teaspoons coconut oil

200 g (7 oz) pork tenderloin, cut into four medallions

100 g (scant ½ cup) cream

1 tablespoon wholegrain Dijon mustard

salt and pepper

Serves: 2

Preparation: approx. 25 minutes

Per portion: approx. 540 kcal, 31 g protein, 44 g fat, 5 g carbohydrate

Put the clarified butter in a pan over a medium heat. Sauté the Savoy cabbage strips and bacon for 2 minutes. Add the mushrooms and continue cooking for a further 2 minutes. Pour in the vegetable stock and season with a pinch each of freshly grated nutmeg, salt and pepper. Cover and simmer over a low heat for about 15 minutes.

Add the coconut oil to a pan over a medium heat. Press the pork medallions slightly flat with the palm of your hand, season with salt and pepper and fry for 3 minutes on each side. Remove, transfer to a plate and cover with foil to keep warm.

Deglaze the pan with the cream, stir in the mustard and bring to the boil. Season to taste with salt and pepper. Place the medallions in the sauce and let infuse for 2 minutes.

In the meantime, season the savoy cabbage and mushroom mixture once more with salt, pepper and nutmeg and divide between two plates. Arrange the medallions on top and serve with the sauce.

TRY WITH KALE

Try this recipe using kale, if you like it. This hearty variety of cabbage almost tastes better here and can be prepared in exactly the same way as the Savoy cabbage.

CHICKEN LEGS IN BACON SAUCE
WITH SAVOY CABBAGE

FOR THE CHICKEN LEGS
AND SAUCE
2 chicken legs
4 teaspoons coconut oil
2 rashers bacon, finely chopped
1 onion, finely diced
100 g (3½ oz) mushrooms, quartered
1 teaspoon tomato purée
50 ml (¼ cup) red wine
200 ml (¾ cup) vegetable stock
½ teaspoon dried thyme
50 g (¼ cup) cream
salt and pepper

FOR THE SAVOY CABBAGE
8 teaspoons butter
200 g (7 oz) savoy cabbage, thinly sliced
freshly grated nutmeg
salt

Serves 2
Preparation: approx. 25 minutes
Cooking: approx. 40 minutes
Per portion: approx. 670 kcal, 34 g
protein, 55 g fat, 5 g carbohydrate

Season the chicken legs with salt and pepper. Add the coconut oil to a pan over a medium heat and fry the chicken legs for 5 minutes until golden brown all over. Transfer them to a 26 × 20 cm (10 × 8 in) baking dish and preheat the oven to 200°C (400°F).

Fry the bacon in the hot chicken pan for 3–4 minutes, stirring occasionally. Add the onion to the bacon in the pan. Add the mushrooms to the pan and continue frying briskly for 3–5 minutes until they are golden brown.

Stir in the tomato purée followed by the red wine. Add the vegetable stock and thyme. Pour the juices over the chicken legs in the baking dish. Transfer the dish to the centre of the oven and bake the chicken for 20 minutes. Turn the chicken legs and continue cooking for 20 minutes.

Heat the butter in a pan and sauté the Savoy cabbage for 2 minutes, stirring occasionally, until it has acquired a bit of colour. Add 3–4 tablespoons of water, season with a generous pinch of salt and freshly grated nutmeg, cover and cook over a low heat for 15 minutes.

Remove the chicken legs from the oven, wrap in foil and keep warm in the switched-off oven.

Transfer the bacon mixture to a pan and pour in the cream. Reduce over a high heat for 6–8 minutes until the sauce has thickened, then season with a pinch of salt.

Season the Savoy cabbage to taste again with salt, arrange on two plates, place the chicken legs on top and serve with the sauce.

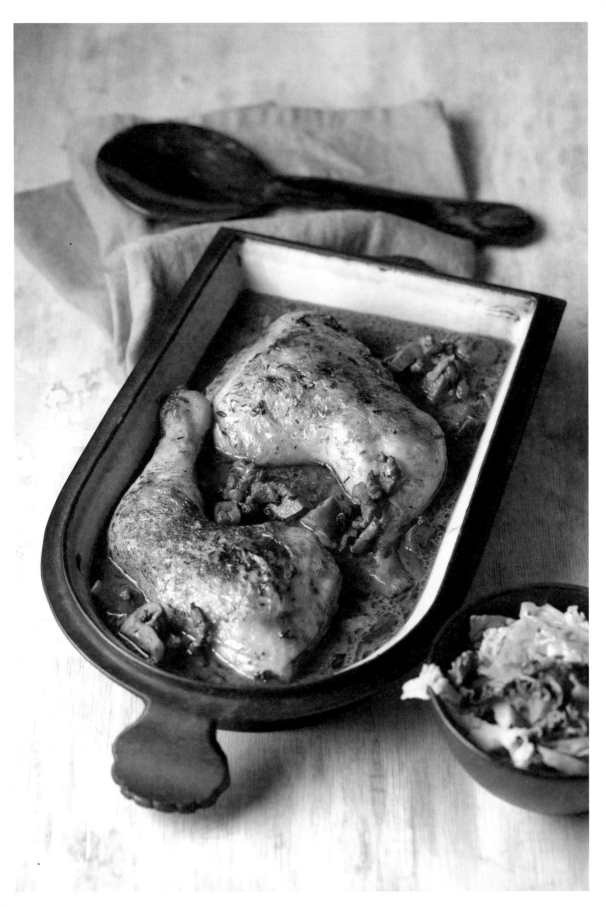

MARINATED PORK NECK STEAKS WITH STAR ANISE

FOR THE STEAKS

1 star anise
½ teaspoon black peppercorns
pinch of ground cinnamon
2 pinches of ground ginger
1 teaspoon medium-hot mustard
3 tablespoons olive oil
zest and juice of ½ orange
2 pork neck steaks (100 g/3½ oz each)
3 teaspoons coconut oil
salt

FOR THE VEGETABLES

4 teaspoons butter
2 yellow pepper, slices into 2 cm
    (¾ in) cubes
50 g (⅓ cup) frozen peas
salt

Serves 2
Preparation: approx. 20 minutes
Marinating: approx. 1 hour
Per portion: 525 kcal, 20 g protein,
45 g fat, 9 g carbohydrate

Crush the star anise and peppercorns together using a pestle and mortar until finely ground. Stir these in a bowl with the cinnamon, ground ginger, mustard, olive oil, ½ teaspoon of salt and the orange zest and juice. Marinate the pork steaks in this mixture, covered in the fridge for at least 1 hour but ideally overnight.

Put the butter in a pan over a medium heat and sauté the peppers, uncovered, for 2 minutes. Add the frozen peas and continue cooking for 3 minutes.

Meanwhile, add the coconut oil to a pan over a medium heat. Take the steaks out of their marinade and let them drain slightly. Fry each one for 3 minutes on each side.

Season the vegetables to taste with salt and divide between two plates. Arrange the steaks on top and serve.

RIBEYE STEAK WITH SAUERKRAUT AND CREAMY CABBAGE

FOR THE CREAMY CABBAGE

300 g (10½ oz) sauerkraut
4 teaspoons butter
50 g (1¾ oz) celeriac, peeled and roughly
    grated
100 ml (scant ½ cup) vegetable stock
50 g (¼ cup) cream
2 juniper berries, crushed or finely
    chopped
1 bay leaf
½ teaspoon dried thyme
½ teaspoon mild ground paprika
salt

FOR THE STEAKS

2 ribeye steaks (approx. 150 g/5 oz each)
3 teaspoons coconut oil
salt and pepper

Serves 2
Preparation: approx. 30 minutes
Per portion: approx. 560 kcal,
    29 g P, 47 g F, 2 g CH

Toss the sauerkraut through with a fork. Put the butter in a pan over a medium heat and sweat the grated celeriac for 3 minutes. Add the sauerkraut and pour in the stock and cream.

Add the juniper berries to the sauerkraut along with the bay leaf, thyme, ground paprika and a pinch of salt, cover and cook over a low heat for 20 minutes.

Just before the sauerkraut is ready, season the steaks on both sides with salt and pepper. Add the coconut oil to a pan over a high heat. Put the steaks in the pan, reduce to a medium heat and fry for 3 minutes on each side. Remove the steaks from the pan, wrap them in foil and let it rest for 5 minutes.

Meanwhile, remove the lid from the sauerkraut and let it bubble over a high heat until the liquid has begun to reduce to a thicker, creamy consistency. Remove the bay leaf and serve the creamy cabbage on two plates with the steaks next to it.

BAKED LEEKS WITH MUSHROOM GRATIN

(V)

1 large leek, halved lengthways and
    sliced into 5–6-cm (2-in) long
    sections
4 teaspoons butter, plus extra
    for greasing
300 g (3⅓ cups) button mushrooms,
    halved or quartered
100 g (scant ½ cup) cream
100 g (3½ oz) Gouda, roughly grated
½ teaspoon dried thyme
freshly grated nutmeg
sprig of thyme, roughly chopped
salt and pepper

Serves 2
Preparation: approx. 20 minutes
Cooking: approx. 30 minutes
Per portion: approx. 400 kcal,
21 g protein, 33 g fat, 5 g carbohydrate

Preheat the oven to 180°C (350°F) and grease a 26 × 20 cm (10 × 8 in) baking dish. Place the leek pieces in the baking dish with the cut surface facing up.

Add the butter to a pan over a high heat and sauté the mushrooms for 2 minutes.

Pour in the cream, bring to the boil, uncovered and simmer for 1 minute over a medium heat. Stir the Gouda swiftly into the cream. Add the dried thyme, season everything with nutmeg, salt and pepper, and pour evenly over the leeks.

Bake the leeks in the centre of the oven for 30 minutes. Arrange the leeks on two plates, garnish with thyme and serve.

FOR A MEATY ALTERNATIVE

Of course, you can use any kind of edible mushroom in this dish, whatever you fancy. It is also delicious with 1–2 tablespoons of chopped ham or bacon added to the recipe, frying it in butter along with the mushrooms. This will give the mushroom sauce a really hearty flavour.

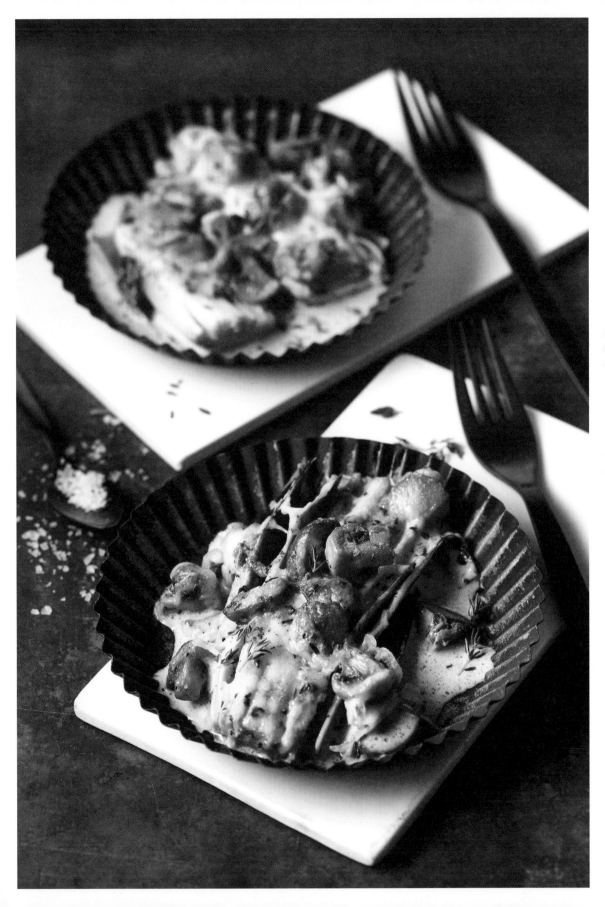

BRAISED PORK BELLY
WITH CELERIAC MASH

FOR THE PORK BELLY
1 small onion, sliced
200 g (7 oz) pork belly (boneless)
¼ teaspoon ground cinnamon
½ teaspoon ground coriander
1 teaspoon ground cumin
1 garlic clove, finely chopped or crushed
250 ml (1 cup) meat stock
salt and pepper

FOR THE CELERIAC MASH
250 g (9 oz) celeriac, peeled and diced
4 teaspoons butter
60 g (generous ¼ cup) cream
freshly grated nutmeg
salt and pepper

Serves 2
Preparation: approx. 25 minutes
Cooking: approx. 1 hour
Per portion: approx. 465 kcal, 21 g
protein, 40 g fat, 5 g carbohydrate

Preheat the oven to 180°C (350°F). Place the onion in a
20-cm (8-in) square baking dish. Using a knife, score five or six
incisions in the skin of the pork belly. Lay it skin-side down on
the onion and season with salt and pepper. Transfer to the
centre of the oven and bake for 15 minutes.

Stir the cinnamon, coriander, cumin and garlic into the meat
stock. Turn the pork belly so the skin is facing up and pour over
the stock. Cook in the oven for a further 45 minutes, using a
ladle to occasionally spoon some of the juices over the meat.
Increase the oven temperature to 225°C (450°F) for the
final 15 minutes.

Cover the celeriac with water in a saucepan, season with salt and
cook for 20 minutes until soft, then drain.

Heat the butter and cream in a small pan and add a pinch of
nutmeg. Add the celeriac, warm briefly and process with a hand
blender to make a creamy purée. Season to taste.

Serve the purée on two plates. Remove the pork belly from the
oven, cut crossways into eight thin slices and arrange these
alongside the celeriac mash. Season the juices to taste with salt
and pepper to serve.

TRY BRAISED NECK OF PORK

You could replace the pork belly with the same quantity of
pork neck. Prepare the meat in the same way as the pork belly.
Then add 1 tablespoon of coconut oil to a pan over a medium
heat. Season the pork neck with salt and pepper and fry it for
3 minutes on each side. Arrange the onions in the baking
dish, lay the neck of pork on top and proceed as described
in the recipe.

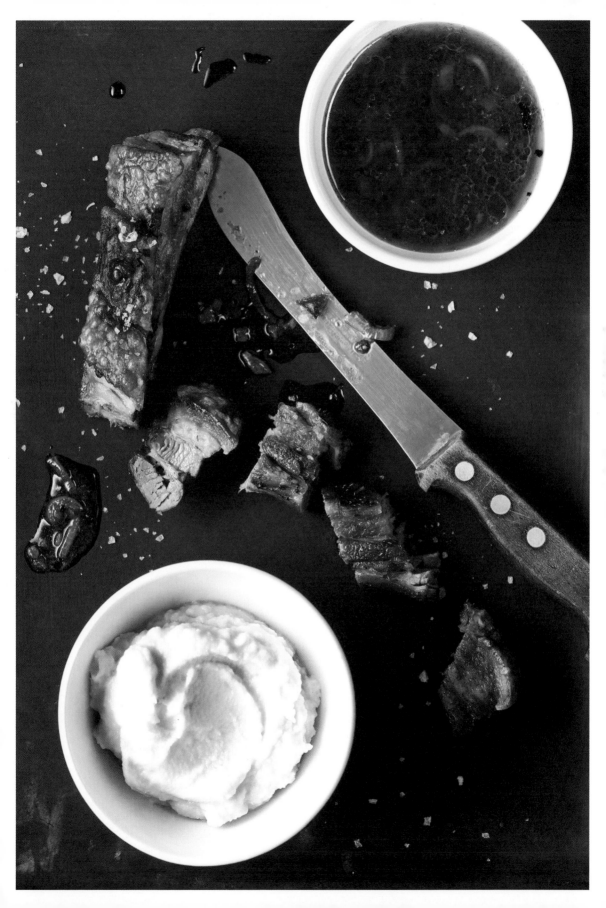

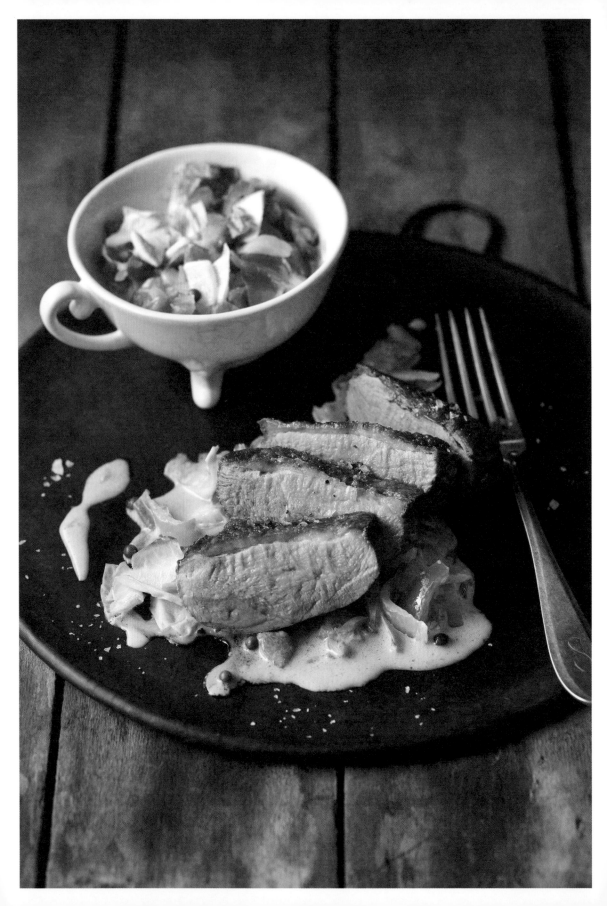

DUCK BREAST ON
A BED OF CHICORY

200 g (7 oz) Barbary duck breast
4 teaspoons clarified butter
1 small red onion, finely diced
2 tomatoes, diced
2 chicory, halved and sliced into roughly
    1 cm (½ in) strips
100 g (scant ½ cup) cream
1 teaspoon green peppercorns in brine
salt and pepper

Serves 2
Preparation: approx. 25 minutes
Per portion: approx. 445 kcal, 21 g
protein, 36 g fat, 7 g carbohydrate

Using a sharp knife, score five or six slight incisions in the skin of the duck breast. Season the skin with salt and pepper.

Add the clarified butter to a pan over a medium heat. Place the duck breast in the pan, skin-side down, and fry for 8 minutes. Season the meat side with salt and pepper, turn the duck breast over and continue frying skin-side up for a further 6 minutes. Remove the duck breast, wrap in foil and let it rest for 8 minutes.

Meanwhile, sauté the onion in the duck fat for 1 minute. Stir in the diced tomato and the chicory, then pour in the cream. Add the green peppercorns with a bit of brine and simmer everything over a high heat, stirring occasionally, until the liquid has reduced to a creamy sauce. Remove from the heat immediately, season generously and transfer to two plates.

Carve the duck breast into 10–12 slices and arrange these on the chicory to serve.

TRY WITH CHINESE CABBAGE

Although chicory has its fans, some people are not so keen on its slightly bitter flavour. If this bitter leaf is not one of your favourite vegetables, just replace it with ½ head of Chinese cabbage. You could also try replacing the green peppercorns with 1 teaspoon of capers. This gives the dish a very different, but equally delicious, flavour.

HALLOUMI WITH PAPAYA
AND TOMATO SALSA

(V)

FOR THE COURGETTE SALAD
1 small courgette
1 tablespoon white wine vinegar
½ teaspoon medium-hot mustard
3 teaspoons olive oil
½ teaspoon dried thyme
salt and pepper

FOR THE SALSA
1 tomato, cubed
½ small papaya, deseeded and finely
    diced
1 small red onion, finely diced
1 mild red chilli, deseeded and
    finely diced
4 basil leaves, sliced into thin strips
1 teaspoons ajvar
salt and pepper

FOR THE HALLOUMI
3 tablespoons olive oil
150 g (5 oz) halloumi

Serves 2
Preparation: approx. 30 minutes
Per portion: approx. 515 kcal,
19 g protein, 43 g fat, 7 g carbohydrate

To make the courgette salad, first wash the courgette, trim off the ends and grate roughly. Toss in the white wine vinegar, mustard, olive oil and thyme. Season to taste with salt and pepper, cover and let infuse in the fridge.

For the salsa, mix the tomato, papaya, red onion, chilli and basil well in the ajvar and season with salt and pepper.

Put the olive oil for the halloumi into a non-stick pan over a medium heat. Cut the halloumi into two equally thick slices and fry these for 2 minutes on both sides until golden brown.

Divide the courgette salad between two plates, arrange the halloumi on top and serve with the papaya and tomato salsa.

COURGETTE AND HALLOUMI KEBABS

To make these, first slice 1 small courgette in half lengthways then cut it into 2 cm (¾ in) chunks. Chop 150 g (5 oz) halloumi into similar bitesize pieces and slide these alternately onto two wooden skewers with the courgette pieces. Heat 2 tablespoons olive oil in a non-stick pan and fry each skewer for 1 minute on each side.

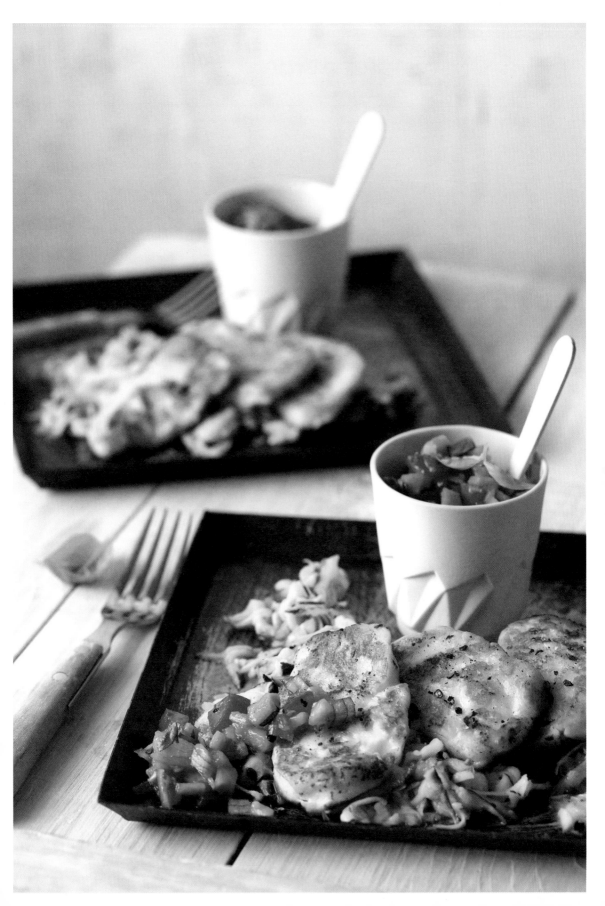

CAULIFLOWER RISOTTO

600 g (1 lb 5 oz) cauliflower florets
150 g (⅔ cup) cream
4 teaspoons butter
1 small onion, finely diced
1 teaspoon curry powder
200 ml (¾ cup) vegetable stock
2 tablespoons flaked almonds
1 tablespoon almond nut butter
20 g (¾ oz) Parmesan, finely grated
3 sprigs of parsley, finely chopped
salt and pepper

Serves 2
Preparation: approx. 30 minutes
Per portion: approx. 600 kcal, 21 g
protein, 50 g fat, 16 g carbohydrate

Bring 500 ml (2 cups) of water to the boil in a pan and add salt. Add a quarter of the cauliflower florets to the pan, cover and cook for 10 minutes before draining in a sieve and transferring to a blender. Add the cream and process everything to a fine purée.

Blitz the remaining cauliflower florets in a food processor until you have crumbs resembling grains of rice. Add the butter to a shallow pan over a medium heat and sauté the onion for 3 minutes. Then add the cauliflower crumbs and continue frying for 1 minute, stirring in the curry powder as you go. Pour in the vegetable stock, cover and cook over the very lowest heat for 5 minutes.

Meanwhile, dry-toast the flaked almonds in a non-stick pan until golden and aromatic.

Add the cauliflower purée, almond nut butter and three quarters of the Parmesan to the cauliflower in the pan. Stir everything well and heat through for 2 minutes. Season to taste with salt and pepper.

Divide between two deep plates, garnished with flaked almonds, parsley and the remaining Parmesan.

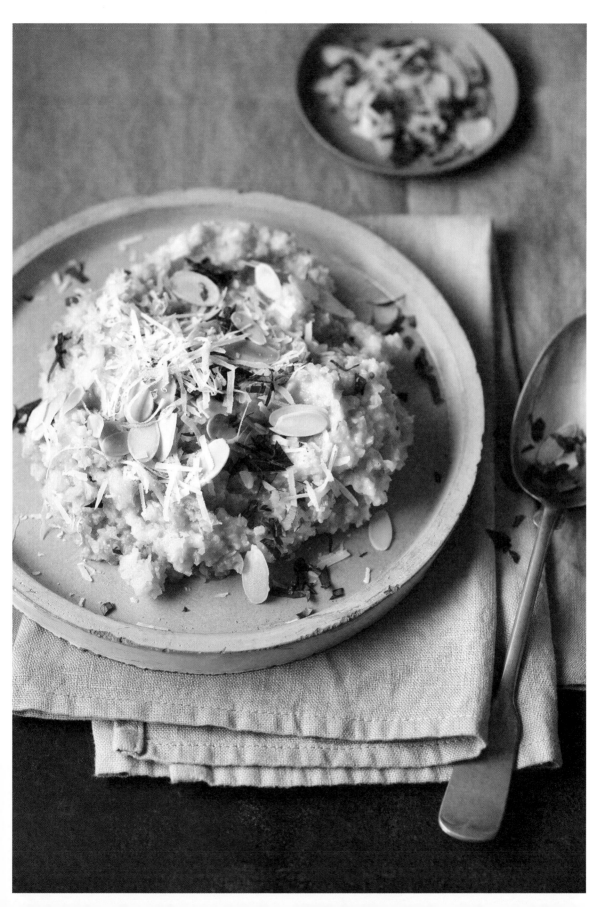

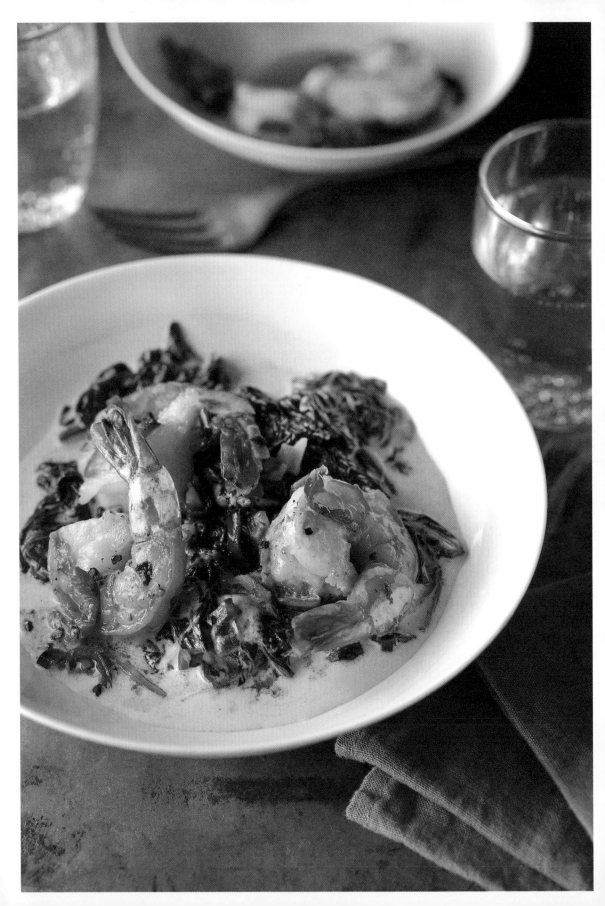

LEMON PRAWNS
ON CREAMED SPINACH

FOR THE SPINACH

4 teaspoons butter

300 g (10½ oz) frozen spinach, defrosted

100 g (scant ½ cup) cream

freshly grated nutmeg

salt

FOR THE PRAWNS

3 teaspoons coconut oil

250 g (9 oz) raw frozen king prawns
    (peeled), defrosted

1 garlic clove, finely chopped or crushed

1 mild red chilli, sliced into thin rings

zest and juice of 1 lemon

salt and pepper

Serves 2

Preparation: approx. 20 minutes

Defrosting: approx. 2 hours

Per portion: approx. 425 kcal, 29 g
protein, 34 g fat, 3 g carbohydrate

Heat the butter for the spinach in a pan. Squeeze all the liquid out of the spinach, roughly chop and sauté for 2 minutes in the butter. Pour in the cream, season with a pinch of salt and nutmeg and cook, uncovered, for 4 minutes over a medium heat.

Meanwhile, add the coconut oil to a non-stick pan over a high heat. Season the prawns with salt and pepper. Fry them for 3 minutes on each side. Add the garlic and chilli as they cook. Finally, deglaze the pan with the lemon juice. Adjust to taste with some grated lemon zest, salt and pepper.

Arrange the spinach on two plates, place the prawns on top, drizzle with the juices and serve.

GENTLE DEFROSTING

It takes quite a while for prawns and spinach to defrost. The best approach is to defrost them both overnight in the fridge, or for about 2 hours at room temperature. But if you're really in a hurry, the spinach can be defrosted with a bit of water in a pan over a low heat, as per the instructions on the pack, and the prawns can be immersed in hot water for 4–5 minutes. Once defrosted, let them drain well and proceed as described above.

SEA BREAM
ON GREEN ASPARAGUS

FOR THE ASPARAGUS
8 teaspoons butter
100 ml (scant ½ cup) vegetable stock
400 g (14 oz) green asparagus, sliced
    into 5 cm (2 in) pieces
freshly grated nutmeg
salt and pepper

FOR THE SEA BREAM
2 sea bream fillets, skin on (approx.
    100 g/3½ oz each)
1 tablespoon coconut oil
salt and pepper

FOR THE TOMATO SAUCE
2 tablespoons coconut oil
1 small onion, finely diced
1 celery stalk, finely diced
100 g (3½ oz) passata (from a jar)
1 teaspoon mild ground paprika
salt and pepper

Serves 2
Preparation: approx. 25 minutes
Per portion: approx. 430 kcal, 24 g
protein, 34 g fat, 7 g carbohydrate

Heat the butter and vegetable stock in a shallow pan. Season with nutmeg, salt and pepper and bring to the boil. Add the asparagus, cover and cook over a low heat for 15 minutes.

Meanwhile, season the skin side of the sea bream fillets with salt and pepper. Add the coconut oil to a pan over a medium heat. Fry the sea bream fillets skin side down for 1 minute, remove from the pan and set aside.

For the tomato sauce, add the coconut oil and diced onion to a pan and sauté for 2 minutes. Then add the celery and continue frying for 2 minutes. Pour in the passata, bring to the boil and simmer for 3–4 minutes. Add the ground paprika and season with salt and pepper.

Place the sea bream fillets, skin side up in the sauce and cook for 2 minutes until done.

Arrange the asparagus on two plates. Place the sea bream fillets on top and serve with the tomato sauce.

BUYING SEA BREAM
Help preserve natural fish stocks by opting for farmed sea bream. Another benefit: thanks to the special food given to farmed bream, they are rich in omega-3 fatty acids with proportionately fewer omega-6 fatty acids. Omega-3 levels can be double those found in wild sea bream!

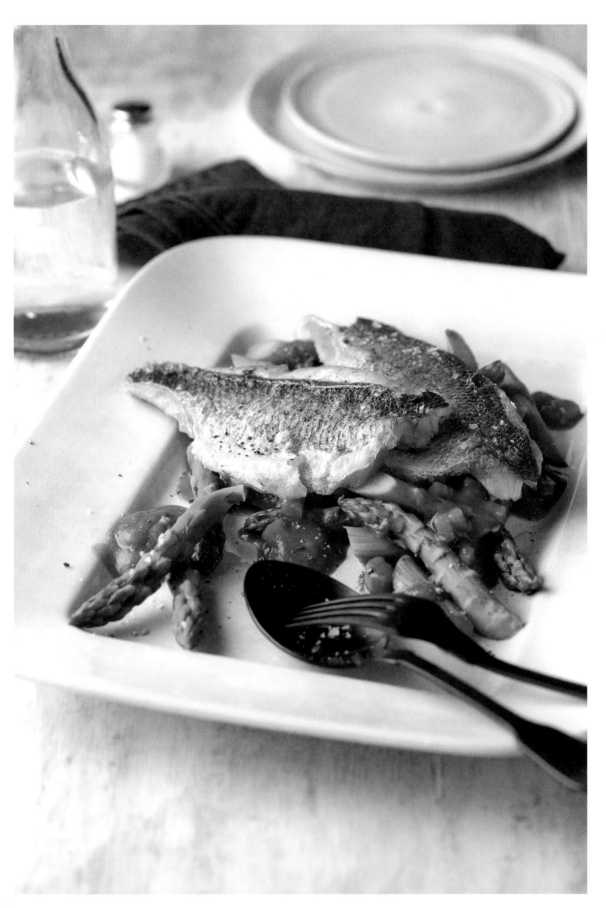

SQUID WITH PAPAYA SALSA

FOR THE SALSA

½ small papaya, peeled, deseeded and
   cubed
1 small red onion, finely diced
1 mild red chilli, sliced into very thin
   rings
juice of ½ lemon
¼ apple, grated
4 teaspoons rapeseed oil
salt and pepper

FOR THE SQUID

4 teaspoons butter
1 garlic clove, finely chopped or crushed
300 g (10½ oz) frozen spinach, defrosted
freshly grated nutmeg
4 teaspoons coconut oil
200 g (7 oz) raw frozen squid tubes
   (ready prepared), defrosted and
   sliced into 1-cm (½-in) wide rings
salt and pepper

Serves 2
Preparation: approx. 20 minutes
Defrosting: approx. 2 hours
Per portion: approx. 415 kcal, 22 g
protein, 30 g fat, 7 g carbohydrate

Stir together the papaya, onion, chilli, lemon juice, apple and rapeseed oil. Season to taste with salt and pepper.

Heat the butter in a pan and sweat the garlic for 1 minute. Squeeze the spinach slightly and add to the pan. Season with a pinch of nutmeg, salt and pepper. Cover and cook over a low heat for 5 minutes.

Add the coconut oil to a pan over a high heat. Season the squid rings with salt and pepper and sauté them for 2–3 minutes, stirring constantly.

Divide the spinach between two plates, arrange the squid rings on top and serve with the papaya salsa.

TENDER SQUID

Squid can easily become tough when cooked. The freezing process helps make the frozen product more tender to start with. If using fresh squid, it's best to bash them before cooking, as you would with schnitzel. For roasting, grilling or frying the trick is speed and heat. For boiling, stewing or braising I recommend lower temperatures and similarly short cooking times to avoid the squid developing a rubbery consistency.

REDFISH ON COURGETTE SPAGHETTI

FOR THE COURGETTE SPAGHETTI

2 courgettes, spiralized (or peeled into tagliatelle-style strips)
3 tablespoons olive oil
1 small onion, finely sliced
salt and pepper

FOR THE REDFISH

8 teaspoons butter
2 redfish fillets (approx. 100 g/3½ oz each)
2 tablespoons flaked almonds
½ teaspoon dried thyme
salt and pepper

Serves 2
Preparation: approx. 20 minutes
Per portion: approx. 515 kcal, 25 g protein, 44 g fat, 5 g carbohydrate

Add the courgette spaghetti to a bowl with ½ teaspoon salt and carefully toss with your hands. Leave for 10 minutes to draw out the water, then transfer to a sieve to drain.

Put the olive oil in a pan over a medium heat and sauté the onion for 1–2 minutes until it has coloured slightly. Add the courgette and continue cooking, uncovered and stirring occasionally, for 3–4 minutes.

Heat the butter in a non-stick pan. Season the redfish fillets with salt and pepper. Fry the fish for 2 minutes on each side, then remove from the pan.

Season the courgette to taste with salt and pepper and serve on two plates. Arrange the redfish fillets on top. Add the flaked almonds and thyme to the butter in the pan and stir. Drizzle this over the fish to serve.

VEGETABLE SPAGHETTI

You can create spaghetti or tagliatelle using a spiralizer or peeler from other vegetables as well as courgette. Long vegetables such as cucumbers and carrots are ideal, as are round kohlrabi or beetroots. Of course, you could also simply slice or dice the courgettes and sauté them in olive oil – but dishes that are pleasing to the eye somehow taste even better.

MONKFISH IN AN ORANGE
AND PEPPER SAUCE

FOR THE MONKFISH

3 teaspoons coconut oil

1 monkfish fillet (approx. 300 g/10½ oz),
    sliced into 6 equal pieces

1 small onion, finely diced

juice of 1 orange

100 ml (scant ½ cup) vegetable stock

1 teaspoon black peppercorns (or
    ¼ teaspoon ground black pepper)

60 g (generous ¼ cup) cream

salt and pepper

FOR THE SALAD

2 tablespoons white wine vinegar

½ teaspoon mustard

4½ tablespoons olive oil

1 handful rocket, cut into
    bitesize pieces

¼ head iceberg lettuce, thinly sliced

½ radicchio, thinly sliced

salt and pepper

Serves 2

Preparation: approx. 30 minutes

Per portion: approx. 535 kcal, 33 g
protein, 47 g fat, 8 g carbohydrate

Add the oil to a pan over a medium heat, season the monkfish
with salt and pepper and sauté for 1 minute on each side.
Remove and set aside on a plate.

Add the onion to the pan and sauté for 2 minutes. Pour in the
orange juice and vegetable stock and bring to the boil. Roughly
crush the peppercorns using a pestle and mortar, add these to
the stock and simmer, uncovered, over a medium heat for
8–10 minutes.

Meanwhile, stir together the vinegar, mustard and olive oil and
season to taste with salt and pepper.

Stir the cream into the orange and pepper sauce, then reduce
over a high heat until the sauce begins to thicken. Remove from
the hob immediately and season to taste with salt.

Toss the salad with the dressing in a bowl. Heat the monkfish
medallions in the sauce for 1 minute, divide the salad between
two plates, arrange the medallions on top and serve with the
sauce.

TRY WITH ROCKET AND TOMATO SALAD

Cut 1 handful of rocket into bitesized pieces. Add 2 tablespoons
of olive oil to a small pan over a medium heat. Braise 100 g
(⅔ cup) cherry tomatoes, halved, in the hot oil for 5 minutes,
stirring occasionally. Season to taste with salt and pepper, fold
into the rocket and serve straight away with the monkfish.

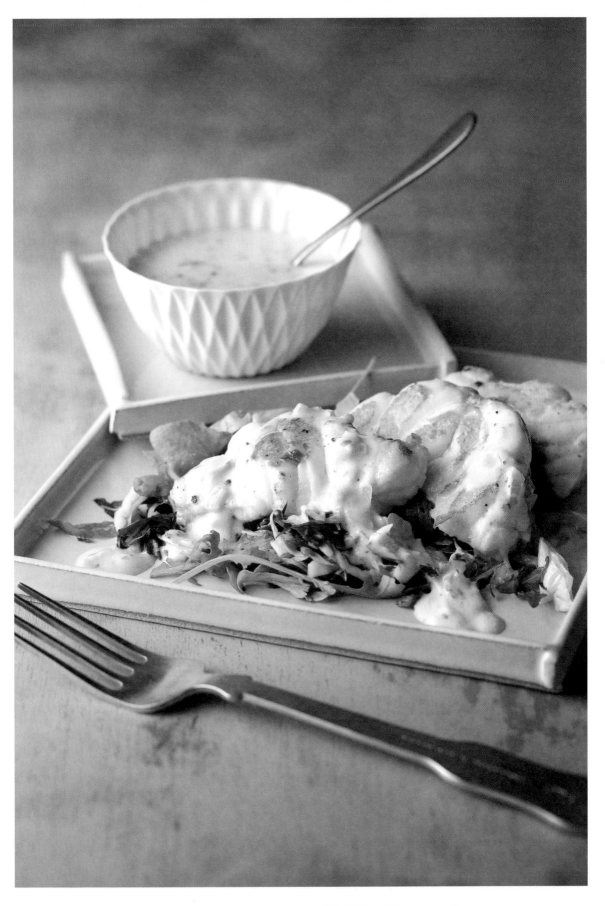

5

SNACKS

You may need a top-up, an emergency bite or just something to keep you going. You can also use these recipes as quick and easy-to-prepare mini meals in place of larger recipes.

MINI AUBERGINE PIZZAS

1 aubergine, cut into 12 × 1½-cm (⅝-in)
thick slices
3 tablespoons olive oil
1 teaspoon oregano
80 g (⅓ cup) chopped tomatoes (tinned)
125 g (4½ oz) ball mozzarella, drained
and sliced into 12 pieces
40 g (1½ oz) goat's cheese
12 basil leaves
salt and pepper

Serves 2
Preparation: approx. 15 minutes
Cooking: approx. 30 minutes
Per portion: approx. 370 kcal, 16 g
protein, 32 g fat, 4 g carbohydrate

Preheat the oven to 200°C (400°F). Line a baking tray with greaseproof paper. Brush the aubergine slices on each side with the olive oil, lay them on the baking tray and season on both sides with a bit of salt. Transfer to the centre of the oven and bake for 20 minutes.

Meanwhile, add the oregano to the tomatoes and season with salt and pepper.

Remove the baked aubergine slices from the oven and spread the tomatoes evenly on top. Add a piece of mozzarella to each one and crumble over the goat's cheese. Continue baking for another 10 minutes.

Remove the 'pizzas' from the oven and garnish each with a basil leaf to serve.

ALTERNATIVE MINI PIZZAS
These pizzas also work brilliantly using kohlrabi or daikon radish, which have strong, aromatic flavours. For this option, peel the kohlrabi or radish, cut it into 6–8 mm (¼–⅜-in) thick slices and cook for about 6 minutes in salted water. Blanch briefly in ice-cold water, dab dry and proceed with the rest of the ingredients as described above.

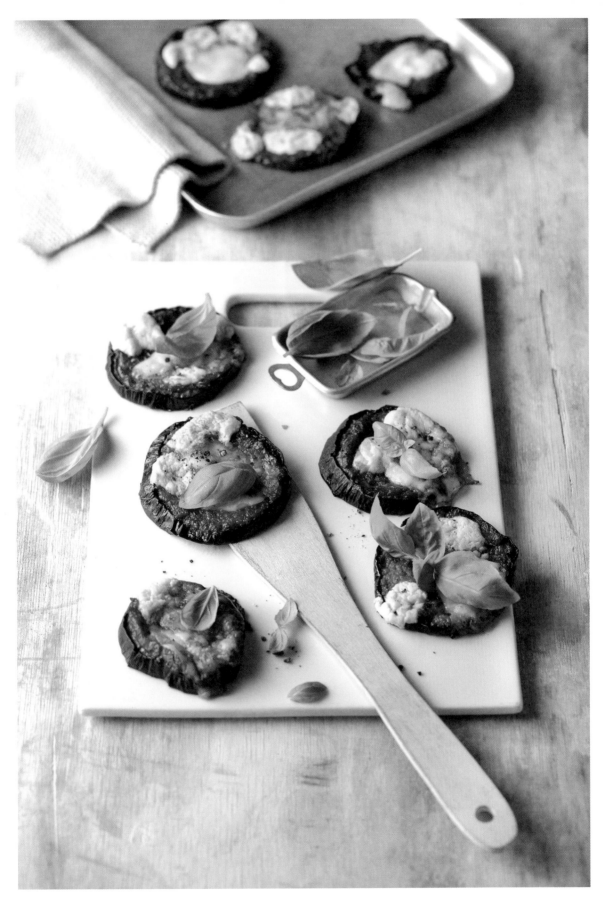

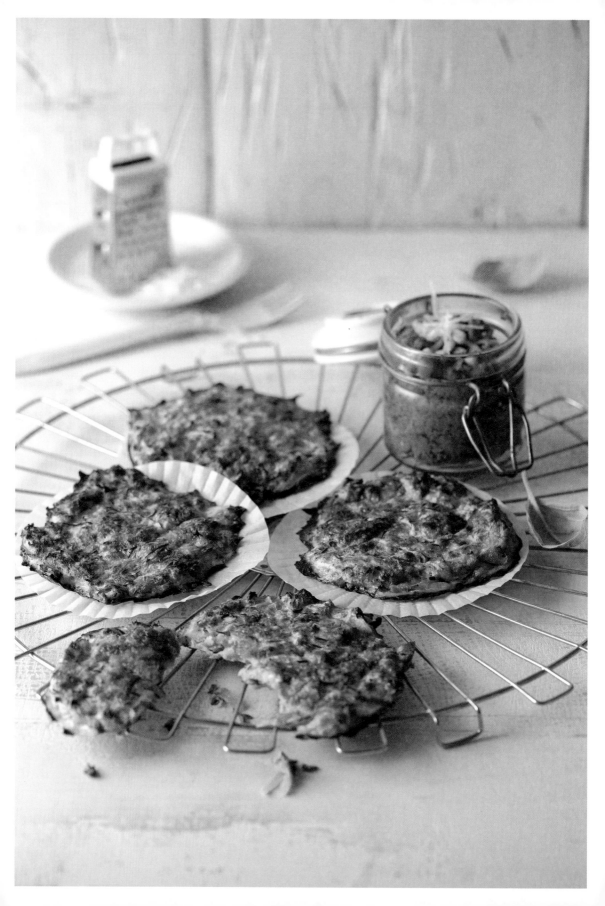

PARMESAN AND COURGETTE PATTIES WITH RED PESTO

(V)

FOR THE PESTO

20 g (2 tablespoons) pine nuts
1 garlic clove, peeled
20 g (¾ oz) Parmesan, finely grated
6 basil leaves
50 g (1¾ oz) dried tomatoes (in oil),
      drained and roughly chopped
4½ tablespoons olive oil
salt and pepper

FOR THE PATTIES

1 courgette (approx. 300 g/10½ oz),
      roughly grated
1 carrot (approx. 100 g/3½ oz), peeled
      and roughly grated
50 g (1¾ oz) Parmesan, roughly grated
1 medium egg
1 teaspoon ground psyllium husks
salt and pepper

Serves 2
Preparation: approx. 25 minutes
Cooking: approx. 20 minutes
Per portion: approx. 590 kcal, 20 g
protein, 53 g fat, 8 g carbohydrate

To make the pesto, toast the pine nuts in a dry pan over a medium heat until they become fragrant. Add the garlic to a blender along with the Parmesan, basil, dried tomatoes, pine nuts and olive oil. Blend to a fine purée. Season to taste with salt and pepper.

Preheat the oven to 400°F. Line a baking tray with baking paper. Squeeze the liquid from the courgette and carrot thoroughly in a clean dish towel. Swiftly mix the vegetables by hand with the Parmesan, egg and ground psyllium husks. Season with a pinch of salt and pepper and let it stand for 5 minutes.

Scoop 10 tablespoons of mixture on the baking tray, spaced slightly apart. Press each one slightly flat. Slide the tray into the centre of the oven and bake the patties for 20 minutes until the edges are golden brown.

Remove from the oven and let the patties cool slightly on the tray for 5 minutes. Arrange on two plates and serve with the pesto.

PESTO FOR THE STORE CUPBOARD

Making just a small quantity of pesto is barely worth the effort. Why not stock up and quadruple the amount? The pesto will keep for several weeks if stored in a sterile jar in the fridge. It also tastes great with a piece of pan-fried or grilled fish.

EASY PEASY
EGG SALAD

6 medium eggs
50 g (3 tablespoons) mayonnaise
50 g (3 tablespoons) Greek yoghurt
3 sprigs of parsley, finely chopped
    (or alternatively 2 teaspoons chopped
    frozen parsley), some reserved
    for garnish
1 teaspoon curry powder
salt and pepper

Serves 2
Preparation: approx. 15 minutes
Per portion: approx. 445 kcal, 20 g
protein, 39 g fat, 3 g carbohydrate

Boil the eggs over a medium heat for 8 minutes to hard-boil. Immerse in cold water and leave to cool.

Stir together the mayonnaise, yoghurt, parsley and curry powder until well combined.

Peel and chop the eggs. Fold the chopped egg into the mayonnaise and yoghurt mixture. Season to taste with salt and pepper, garnish with the reserved parsley and serve.

STUFFED EGGS
WITH BACON

6 medium eggs
3 rashers bacon, finely diced
40 g (2½ tablespoons) mayonnaise
2 dried tomatoes (in oil), drained and
    chopped finely
2 spring onions, sliced into thin rings
salt and pepper

Serves 2
Preparation: approx. 15 minutes
Per portion: approx. 455 kcal, 22 g
protein, 40 g fat, 2 g carbohydrate

Boil the eggs over a medium heat for 8 minutes to hard-boil. Immerse in cold water and leave to cool.

Fry the bacon in a dry pan for 6 minutes until crisp.

Peel the eggs, slice in half lengthways and scoop out the yolk with a teaspoon. Mash the yolk with a fork and stir it together with the mayonnaise, bacon, tomatoes and spring onions. Season to taste with salt and pepper, then use a teaspoon or piping bag to fill the halved and hollowed out eggs with the mixture.

EGG CARPACCIO
WITH DIP

6 medium eggs
juice of ½ lemon
50 g (3 tablespoons) mayonnaise
30 g (2 tablespoons) cream
a bunch of chives, snipped into
    little rings
2 radishes, roughly grated
salt and pepper

Serves 2
Preparation: approx. 25 minutes
Per portion: approx. 465 kcal, 20 g
protein, 41 g fat, 3 g carbohydrate

Boil the eggs over a medium heat for 8 minutes to hard-boil. Immerse in cold water and leave to cool.

Mix the lemon juice with the mayonnaise, cream, chives and radishes. Season to taste with salt and pepper.

Peel the eggs and cut into 5-mm (¼-in) thick slices. Arrange the slices in a fan pattern on two plates. Drizzle with the chive dip to serve.

EGGS BAKED
IN TOMATOES

4 teaspoons coconut oil
6 tomatoes
6 basil leaves
40 g (1½ oz) Parmesan, finely grated
2 medium eggs
2½ tablespoons cream
freshly grated nutmeg
60 g (2 oz) feta, cut into 6 cubes
salt and pepper

Serves 2
Preparation: approx. 15 minutes
Cooking: approx. 25 minutes
Per portion: approx. 385 kcal,
21 g protein, 30 g fat, 6 g carbohydrate

Preheat the oven to 200°C (400°F). Grease a 20-cm (8-in) square baking dish with 1 teaspoon of the oil. Slice a lid off each tomato. Hollow them out, place in the baking dish and insert 1 basil leaf.

Whisk the Parmesan with the eggs, cream and remaining coconut oil. Season with salt, pepper and nutmeg and divide between the tomatoes. Bake in the centre of the oven for 8 minutes.

Place 1 cube of feta on each tomato, then continue baking for a further 13–17 minutes.

KOHLRABI FRIES WITH
STRAWBERRY KETCHUP

(V)

FOR THE KOHLRABI FRIES
3 tablespoons coconut oil, melted
1 teaspoon mild ground paprika
1 teaspoon curry powder
1 large kohlrabi, cut into 8-mm
    (⅜-in) batons
salt and pepper

FOR THE KETCHUP
50 g (⅓ cup) strawberries, hulled
1 tablespoon tomato purée
1 teaspoon white wine vinegar
1 small red chilli, halved and deseeded
salt and pepper

Serves 2
Preparation: approx. 20 minutes
Cooking: approx. 20 minutes
Per portion: approx. 160 kcal, 2 g protein,
15 g fat, 5 g carbohydrate

Preheat the oven to 250°C (440°F). Line a baking tray with greaseproof paper. Stir together the melted coconut oil, ground paprika, curry powder, 1 teaspoon of salt and a pinch of pepper in a bowl. Add the kohlrabi batons and mix well until they are evenly coated.

Spread the kohlrabi fries over the baking tray, making sure they touch each other as little as possible. Slide the tray into the centre of the oven and bake for 20 minutes. Turn the fries after 10 minutes to ensure they brown evenly.

Meanwhile, add the strawberries to a blender with the tomato purée, vinegar and chilli. Blend everything well and season to taste with salt and pepper.

Remove the kohlrabi fries from the oven and serve with the strawberry ketchup.

SUBSTITUTE WITH SQUASH
Try making these fries with a hokkaido squash, or maybe a daikon radish, instead of the kohlrabi. Both are prepared in the same way. These fries are also a fantastic side dish.

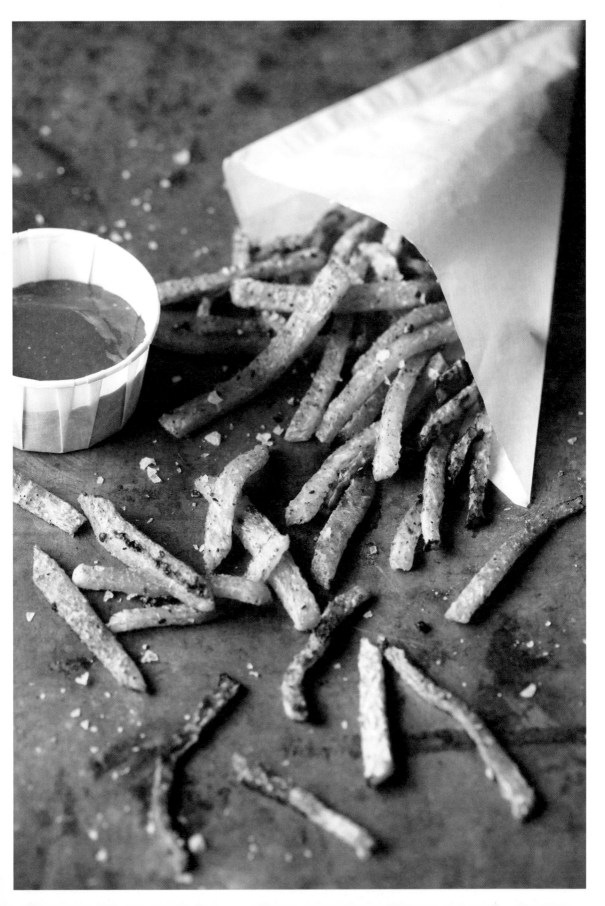

CRISPY COURGETTE
WITH HERB AIOLI

FOR THE AIOLI

1½ teaspoons milk

50 ml (¼ cup) olive oil

1 medium egg yolk

1 garlic clove, roughly chopped

1 tablespoon dried Italian herbs

salt and pepper

FOR THE COURGETTE

1 medium egg

20 g (¾ oz) Parmesan, finely grated

30 g (⅓ cup) ground almonds

1 teaspoon mild paprika

1 teaspoon dried thyme

1 large courgette, sliced into 8-mm
    (⅜-in) thick discs

3 tablespoons coconut oil

salt

Serves 2

Preparation: approx. 20 minutes

Per portion: approx. 580 kcal, 14 g
protein, 57 g fat, 3 g carbohydrate

Peel and roughly chop the garlic. Add the milk, olive oil and egg yolk to a blender. Slowly blend in pulses until the mixture has thickened to form a kind of mayonnaise.

Add the garlic and herbs to the mayonnaise and mix again. Season to taste with salt and pepper.

Whisk the egg in a deep bowl. Mix the Parmesan with the ground almonds, paprika, thyme and a pinch of salt in a second bowl. First dip the courgette slices in the egg, then coat both sides with the almond mixture.

Add the oil to a non-stick pan over a medium heat. Fry the coated courgette slices in the hot oil on each side for 2 minutes until golden brown.

Remove and let drain on kitchen paper before arranging on two plates. Serve with the herb aioli.

AIOLI WITHOUT EGG

If you prefer to avoid raw eggs, there is a simple alternative. If all the ingredients are puréed with a hand blender, they will thicken and combine even without the raw egg yolk. Insert the hand blender into the beaker and only switch it on when it is immersed, then slowly raise and lower it. However, the mixture will only keep its consistency for a few minutes. So, if you choose the egg-free version, it's best to make the aioli right before serving.

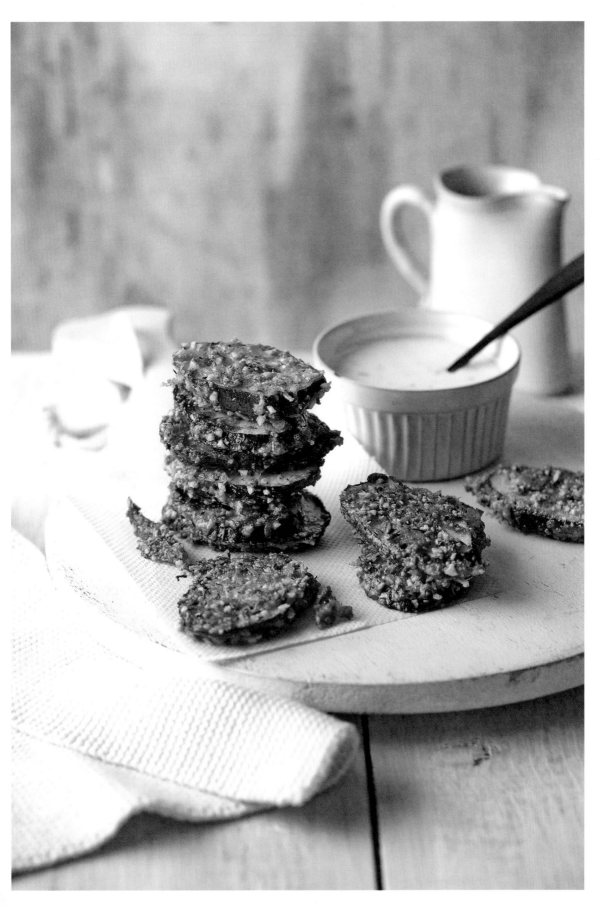

"QUATTRO FORMAGGI" MUFFINS

50 g (⅓ cup) almonds
50 g (⅓ cup) cashew nuts
30 g (1 oz) dried tomatoes (in oil),
    drained
a small bunch of basil, leaves picked
50 g (1¾ oz) Parmesan, finely grated
50 g (1¾ oz) Gouda, roughly grated
50 g (1¾ oz) mozzarella, roughly grated
150 g (heaping ½ cup) quark
    (40 % fat)
4 medium eggs
1 teaspoon baking powder
salt and pepper

Makes 12
Preparation: approx. 25 minutes
Baking: approx. 20 minutes
Per muffin: approx. 170 kcal, 10 g
protein, 13 g fat, 2 g carbohydrate

Preheat the oven to 350°F. Line a 12-hole muffin tin with paper cases.

Finely grind the almonds and cashew nuts in a food processor. Add the dried tomatoes and basil leaves and blitz again to a fine consistency.

Add the cheeses to a bowl along with the nut mixture and quark. Add the eggs and baking powder and combine everything well. Season with salt and pepper and divide the mixture evenly between the muffin cases.

Slide the tray into the centre of the oven and bake for 20 minutes. Remove and leave to cool briefly. Take the muffins out of the tray and serve still warm, or leave them to cool and store in an airtight container.

CHANGE UP THE CHEESE
Why not replace the mozzarella with the same quantity of soft goat's cheese or blue cheese?

BEETROOT CRISPS WITH
SOURED CREAM AND ONION

FOR THE CRISPS
1 beetroot
3 teaspoons olive oil
salt and pepper

FOR THE DIP
1 spring onion, halved lengthways then
    sliced into thin crescents
3 sprigs of parsley, finely chopped (or
    1 tablespoon chopped frozen parsley)
50 g (scant ¼ cup) crème fraîche
1 tablespoon quark (40 % fat)
salt and pepper

Serves 2
Preparation: approx. 15 minutes
Cooking: approx. 40 minutes
Per portion: approx. 215 kcal, 3 g protein,
19 g fat, 8 g carbohydrate

Preheat the oven to 150°C (300°F) on the fan setting. Line a baking tray with greaseproof paper. Peel the beetroot (see below). Using a mandoline or slicer, create very thin rounds from the beetroot (2 mm/⅛ in). Add these to a bowl and mix well with olive oil and a pinch of salt and pepper.

Lay the slices individually on the baking tray. Transfer to the centre of the oven and bake for 20 minutes. Turn them and continue cooking for 20 minutes. During this process, open the oven door briefly every 10 minutes to allow any moisture to escape.

Meanwhile, prepare the dip. In a bowl, stir together the spring onions, parsley, crème fraîche and quark and season to taste with salt and pepper.

After 40 minutes, test whether the beetroot crisps are sufficiently crisp. If not, reduce the oven temperature to 100°C (200°F) and let the crisps dry out for another 20 minutes with the oven door slightly ajar. Serve the crisps in two bowls with the dip alongside.

PREPARING BEETROOT
Beetroot juice produces stubborn stains, so you should ideally wear household gloves when peeling them. You can buy a mandoline for very little money, but if you are really skilled using a knife, you can cut wafer-thin beetroot slices freehand.

LEFTOVERS
Juice any leftover beetroot, or dress with orange and olive oil for a delicious salad.

SPINACH MUFFINS
WITH BACON

3 teaspoons coconut oil
10 rashers bacon, finely chopped
1 small onion, finely diced
1 garlic clove, finely chopped or crushed
200 g (7 oz) frozen spinach, defrosted
5 medium eggs
30 g (¼ cup) coconut flour
1 teaspoon baking powder
freshly grated nutmeg
12 cherry tomatoes, halved
salt and pepper

Makes 12
Preparation: approx. 20 minutes
Baking: approx. 20 minutes
Defrosting: approx. 2 hours
Per muffin: approx. 80 kcal, 5 g protein,
6 g fat, 1 g carbohydrate

Preheat the oven to 180°C (350°F). Line a 12-hole muffin tin with paper cases.

Put the coconut oil in a pan over a medium heat and fry the bacon for about 3 minutes. Add the onion and garlic and continue cooking for another 3 minutes until golden brown.

Meanwhile, squeeze the spinach, chop roughly and mix with the eggs, coconut flour and baking powder. Add the fried onion and bacon mixture, mix and season with salt, pepper and freshly grated nutmeg.

Divide the mixture evenly between the muffin cases. Put two cherry tomato halves on each muffin. Slide the tray into the centre of the oven and bake the muffins for 20 minutes. Remove from the oven and leave to cool briefly. Take the muffins out of the tin and serve while still warm, or leave to cool and store in an airtight container in the fridge.

BREAKFAST MUFFINS WITH SALMON
For Sunday breakfast, you could replace the bacon with the same quantity of smoked salmon. Unlike the bacon, the salmon doesn't need frying. Just dice it finely and fold it into the spinach mixture at the end with the sautéed onion.

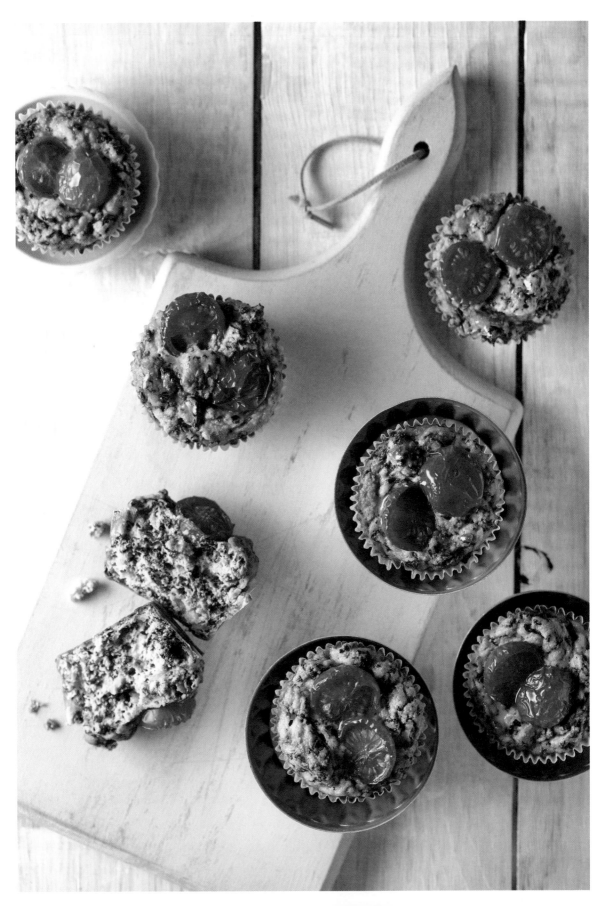

MINI PEPPERS WITH CREAM CHEESE

6 sweet mini peppers
20 g (¾ oz) Parmesan, finely grated
80 g (scant ⅓ cup) full-fat cream cheese
20 g (¼ cup) ground almonds
1 teaspoon dried thyme
6 rashers bacon
salt and pepper

Serves 2
Preparation: approx. 15 minutes
Cooking: approx. 10 minutes
Per portion: approx. 310 kcal, 13 g
protein, 27 g fat, 4 g carbohydrate

Preheat the oven to 200°C (400°F). Line a baking tray with greaseproof paper. Slice a lid off each of the peppers. If necessary, remove any white membrane or seeds.

Combine the Parmesan, cream cheese, ground almonds, and thyme to create the creamy filling. Season to taste with salt and pepper.

Transfer the cream into a piping bag fitted with a round nozzle and fill each pepper up to the rim with this mixture.

Wrap a rasher of bacon lengthways around each pepper so the opening is covered. Fix the bacon in place with a toothpick. Transfer the stuffed peppers to a baking tray and bake in the centre of the oven for 10 minutes. Remove and serve.

FILLING THE PEPPERS

If you don't have a piping bag to hand, you can also use a teaspoon to scoop the cream into the peppers, or you can adapt a freezer bag for this purpose by snipping off a little bit of one corner.

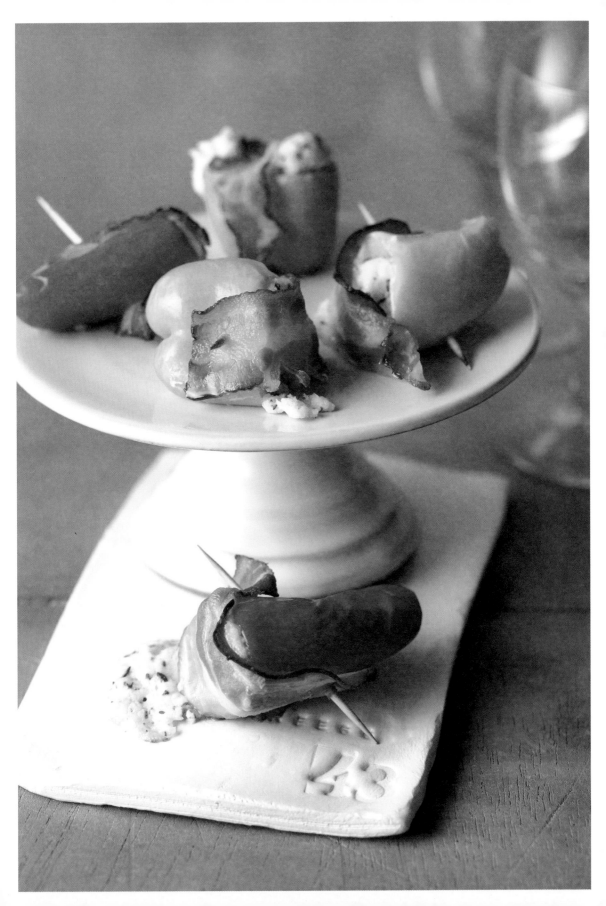

6

SWEET TREATS

We are not fans of sugar, but you can
find sweetness in other places. Dark chocolate
is delicious on its own, but with minimum
70% cocoa solids. Birch sugars are also good
substitutes, but not so much that you are
tempted into too many calories and offset
the keto effect.

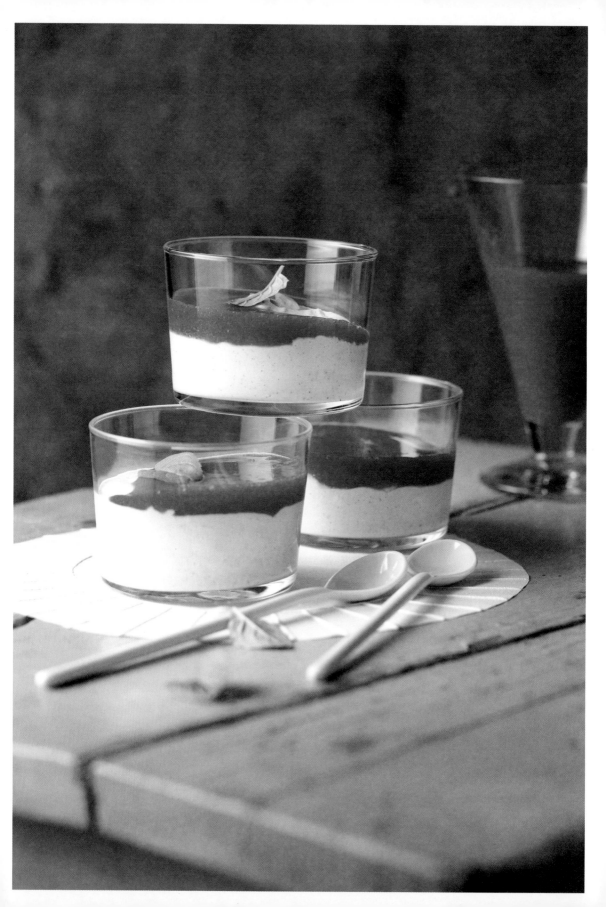

YOGHURT PANNA COTTA
WITH STRAWBERRY SAUCE

FOR THE PANNA COTTA
4 sheets gelatine
1 vanilla pod
150 g (⅔ cup) cream
¼ teaspoon ground cinnamon
200 g (¾ cup) Greek yoghurt
birch sugar (xylitol, optional)

FOR THE STRAWBERRY SAUCE
zest and juice of ½ lime
150 g (1 cup) strawberries, hulled
4 mint leaves, to serve

Serves 2
Preparation: approx. 25 minutes
Chilling: approx. 4 hours
Per portion: approx. 390 kcal, 10 g
protein, 33 g fat, 11 g carbohydrate

Soak the gelatine for 5 minutes in ice-cold water. Meanwhile, slice the vanilla pod lengthways and scrape out the seeds. Add both seeds and pod to a pan with the cream, cinnamon, 50 ml (¼ cup) of water and bring to the boil.

Remove the gelatine from the water and squeeze it out. Stir the gelatine into the hot cream until it has completely dissolved. Remove the vanilla pod, stir in the yoghurt and add birch sugar to taste, if desired. Divide the panna cotta between two glasses or dessert dishes. Cover and chill for at least 4 hours or overnight.

Add the lime zest and juice and strawberries to a blender and blend until smooth. Spread the strawberry purée over the panna cotta and garnish with mint leaves to serve.

TRY WITH CHOCOLATE SAUCE

To make a chocolate sauce instead of the strawberry option, finely chop or grate 40 g (1½ oz) dark chocolate (minimum 70% cocoa content). Bring 100 g (scant ½ cup) cream to the boil in a pan, then remove from the heat. Add the chocolate and stir until it has completely melted. Add ½ teaspoon vanilla powder and birch sugar to taste. Let the chocolate sauce cool completely before serving.

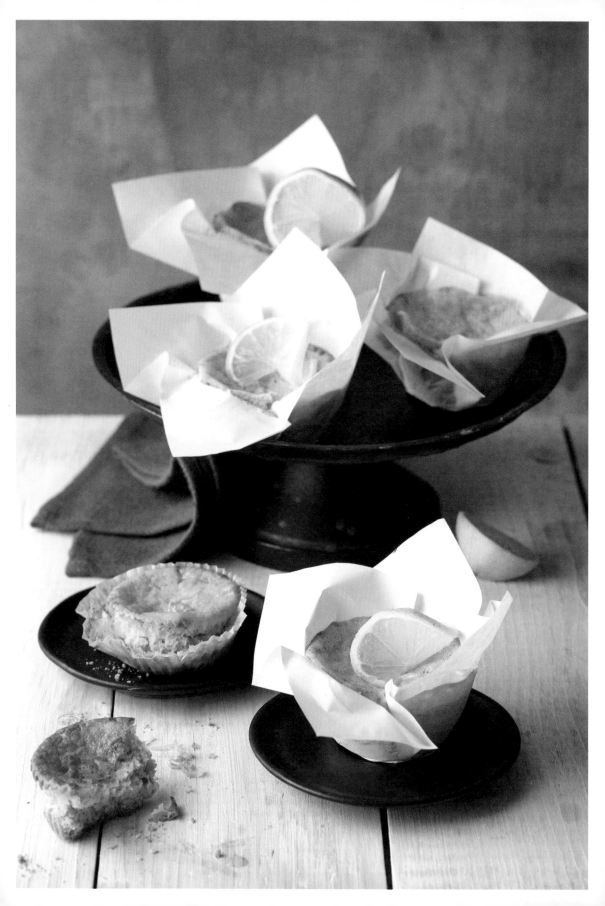

LEMON CREAM CHEESE MUFFINS

FOR THE BASE

90 g (3¼ oz) butter

120 g (1¼ cups) almond flour

salt

FOR THE FILLING

3 medium eggs

300 g (1¼ cups) full-fat cream cheese

2 teaspoons baking powder

½ teaspoon vanilla powder

zest of 1 lemon, plus ½ lemon, very
    thinly sliced to decorate

zest of ½ orange

birch sugar (xylitol, optional)

salt

Makes 12

Preparation: approx. 20 minutes

Baking: approx. 30 minutes

Per muffin: approx. 170 kcal, 7 g protein,
15 g fat, 1 g carbohydrate

Preheat the oven to 340°F. Line a 12-hole muffin tin with paper cases.

Melt the butter and work it into the almond flour with a pinch of salt to create a crumbly consistency. Divide this crumbly mixture evenly between the muffin cases and press down firmly, so the base of each case is covered. Transfer to the centre of the oven and bake for 10 minutes.

Meanwhile, stir together the eggs, cream cheese, baking powder, vanilla powder, a pinch of salt, plus the lemon and orange zest until well combined. Add some birch sugar, if desired.

Pour the mixture onto the pre-baked muffin bases and continue baking in the centre of the oven for 20 minutes. Remove the muffins from the oven, leave to cool briefly, then remove from the tin to cool completely on a wire rack.

Decorate the muffins with the thin lemon slices.

FREEZING THE MUFFINS

These muffins freeze really well if individually protected with plastic wrap. This way you'll always have some supplies. Just defrost the frozen muffins for 10–12 minutes in an oven preheated to 200°C (400°F), or warm up defrosted muffins in the microwave or toaster and enjoy!

LEMON AND YOGHURT JELLIES

8 sheets gelatine
zest and juice of 1 lemon
100 ml (scant ½ cup) apple juice
7 teaspoons olive oil
½ sachet unsweetened powdered
    lemon jelly
100 g (⅓ cup) Greek yoghurt
birch sugar (xylitol, optional)

Makes 20
Preparation: approx. 15 minutes
Chilling: approx. 6 hours
Per gelée: approx. 30 kcal, 1 g protein, 2
g fat, 1 g carbohydrate

Soak the gelatine for 5 minutes in ice-cold water. Mix the lemon juice, apple juice, olive oil and 1 tablespoon of water in a saucepan.

Stir in the powdered jello and bring to the boil, stirring occasionally, then immediately remove from the hob.

Squeeze out the gelatine by hand and dissolve it in the hot liquid. Stir in the yoghurt and lemon zest and some birch sugar to taste, if desired. Divide the mixture evenly into a 20-hole silicone bundt tray.

Chill for at least 6 hours in the fridge until set, ideally overnight. Press out of the silicone moulds and store in an airtight container in the fridge until ready to eat. The yoghurt jellies will keep, chilled, for 1 week.

RASPBERRY YOGHURT GELÉES

Replace the lemon with 100 g (generous ¾ cup) raspberries. Blend the raspberries with 50 ml (¼ cup) apple juice and 50 ml (¼ cup) water, then press them through a sieve to remove the seeds. Stir in ½ sachet unsweetened raspberry jelly and continue as described.

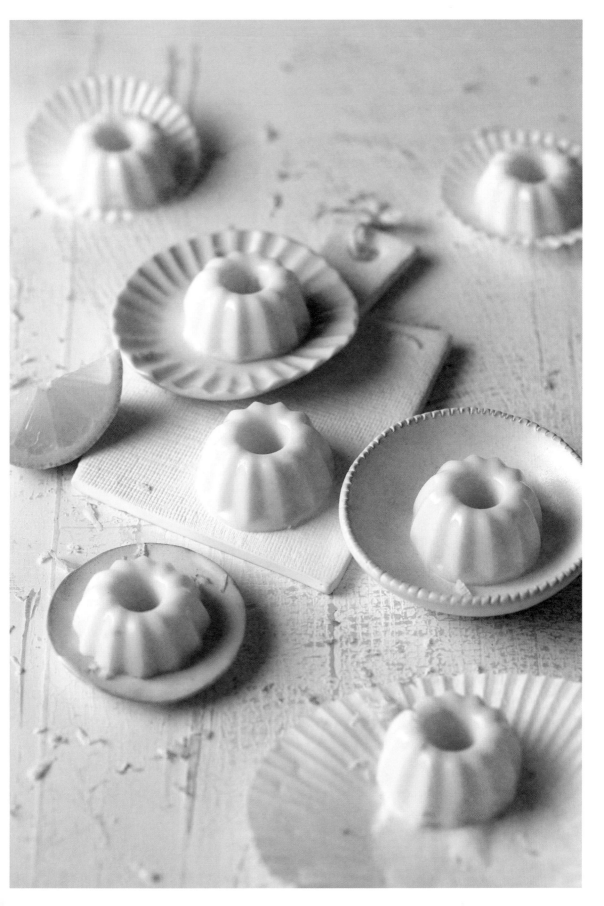

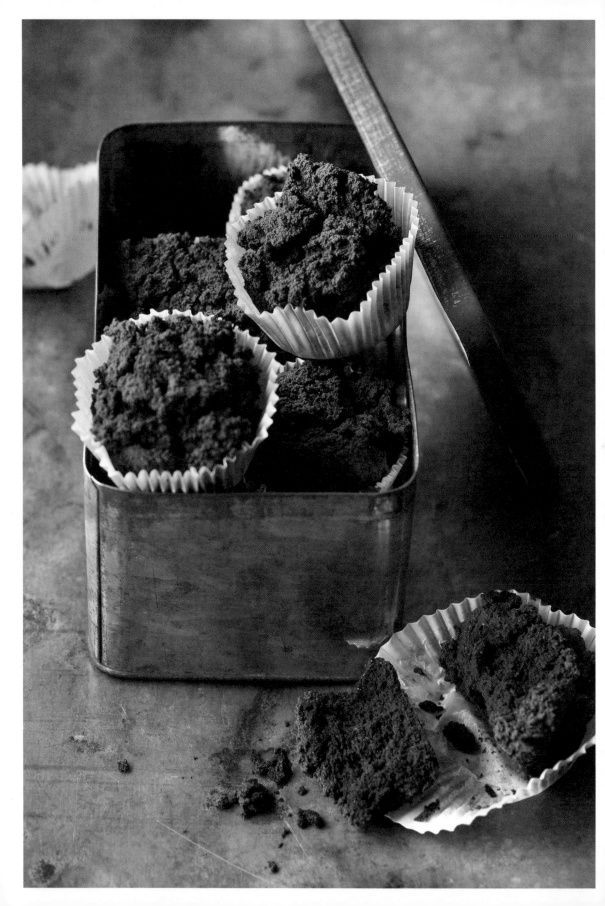

AVOCADO AND CHOCOLATE MUFFINS

180 g (scant 2 cups) almond flour
70 g (heaping ½ cup) cocoa powder
½ teaspoon baking soda
½ teaspoon baking powder
1 avocado, peeled and destoned
4 tablespoons coconut oil, melted
280 g (1 cup) Greek yoghurt
2 medium eggs
½ teaspoon vanilla powder
birch sugar (xylitol, optional)

Makes 12
Preparation: approx. 20 minutes
Baking: approx. 25 minutes
Per muffin: approx. 180 kcal, 9 g protein,
15 g fat, 2 g carbohydrate

Preheat the oven to 350°F. Line a 12-hole muffin tin with paper cases. Combine the almond flour, cocoa powder, baking soda and baking powder and sift into a bowl through a sieve. Scoop the avocado flesh into a blender with the melted coconut oil, yoghurt, eggs and vanilla powder and blend until smooth. Sift the dry ingredients into the avocado mixture.

Stir until everything is well combined. Optionally, add some birch sugar to sweeten, then use a tablespoon to divide the mixture evenly between the muffin cases.

Slide the tray into the centre of the oven and bake for 25 minutes. Remove, leave to cool briefly, then remove the muffins from the tin to cool completely on a wire rack.

TRY WITH DARK CHOCOLATE

Try the recipe with 60 g (2 oz) dark chocolate instead of the cocoa powder; this makes the muffins even more moist. For this version you will need to grate the chocolate as finely as possible. Just fold the chocolate into the mixture right at the end.

CHOCO-NUT BITES

80 g (3 oz) dark chocolate (minimum 70%
　　cocoa content), finely chopped
50 g (½ cup) pecans, roughly chopped
30 g (¼ cup) almonds, roughly chopped
10 g (3½ teaspoons) hulled
　　pumpkin seeds
fleur de sel (or sea salt)

Makes 6
Preparation: approx. 15 minutes
Chilling: approx. 1 hours
Per bite: approx. 165 kcal, 3 g protein, 15
g fat, 5 g carbohydrate

Line a baking tray with greaseproof paper. Melt the chocolate in a little bowl suspended over a bain-marie, stirring occasionally. Add the nuts to the melted chocolate and stir until well-coated.

Scoop six tablespoons of the chocolate and nut mixture to create little heaps, placed slightly apart on the baking tray. Scatter the nutty heaps with pumpkin seeds and sprinkle over a few grains of fleur de sel.

Transfer the choco-nut bites to the fridge for 1 hour until the chocolate has set. They will keep for up to 2 weeks in an airtight container stored in the fridge.

CHOCOLATE COCONUT BALLS

1 avocado, peeled and destoned
100 g (heaping ⅓ cup) full-fat
   cream cheese
50 g (1¾ oz) soft butter
60 g (½ cup) coconut flour
30 g (¼ cup) cocoa powder
½ teaspoon vanilla powder
birch sugar (xylitol, optional)
60 g (heaping ½ cup) ground almonds
20 g (¼ cup) desiccated coconut

Makes 20 balls
Preparation: approx. 20 minutes
Per ball: approx. 90 kcal, 2 g protein,
9 g fat, 1 g carbohydrate

Scoop the avocado flesh into a food processor. Add the cream cheese, butter, coconut flour, cocoa powder and vanilla powder and process everything until well combined. Add some birch sugar, if desired.

Transfer to a bowl, knead in the ground almonds and let it rest for 10 minutes. Shape 20 equal-size balls from the mixture using your hands and toss them in desiccated coconut. The chocolate coconut balls will keep for up to 1 week if stored in an airtight container in the fridge.

A DIFFERENT COATING

Instead of the desiccated coconut, try a handful of roasted, unsalted pistachios – they can be chopped up in no time and ground in a food processor and will be considerably cheaper than raw, ready-shelled pistachio kernels. Another great option for a deliciously different flavour is to use flaked almonds, chopped slightly smaller using a knife.

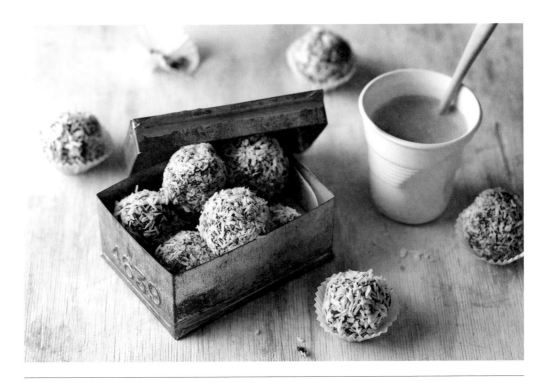

PEANUT BARS

200 g (7 oz) dark chocolate (minimum
    70% cocoa content), finely chopped
4 tablespoons peanut butter
    (unsweetened)
1 tablespoon butter
120 g (¾ cup) salted peanuts,
    roughly chopped
birch sugar (xylitol, optional)

Makes 8 bars
Preparation: approx. 15 minutes
Chilling: approx. 4 hours
Per bar: approx. 295 kcal, 9 g protein,
24 g fat, 10 g carbohydrate

Line a 20 × 16 cm (8 × 6 in) dish with greaseproof paper.
Melt the chocolate in a little bowl over a bain-marie, stirring
occasionally.

Combine the peanut butter with the chocolate, then stir in the
butter until it has completely melted. Finally, fold in the peanuts
until well mixed. Add some birch sugar, if desired.

Spoon into the dish, smooth the surface and chill in the fridge for
at least 4 hours, ideally overnight.

Use the greaseproof paper to lift the solid chocolate block out of
the dish, transfer to a chopping board and slice into eight bars,
measuring roughly 8 × 3 cm (3 × 1 in). The bars will keep, chilled
in an airtight container, for up to 4 weeks.

BETTER WITHOUT SWEETENERS

If sweetened, these bars are so tempting – you can easily polish
off too many and slip out of ketosis. So it's best to not add any
sweeteners, or only make a batch when you are certain you'll be
able to resist them.

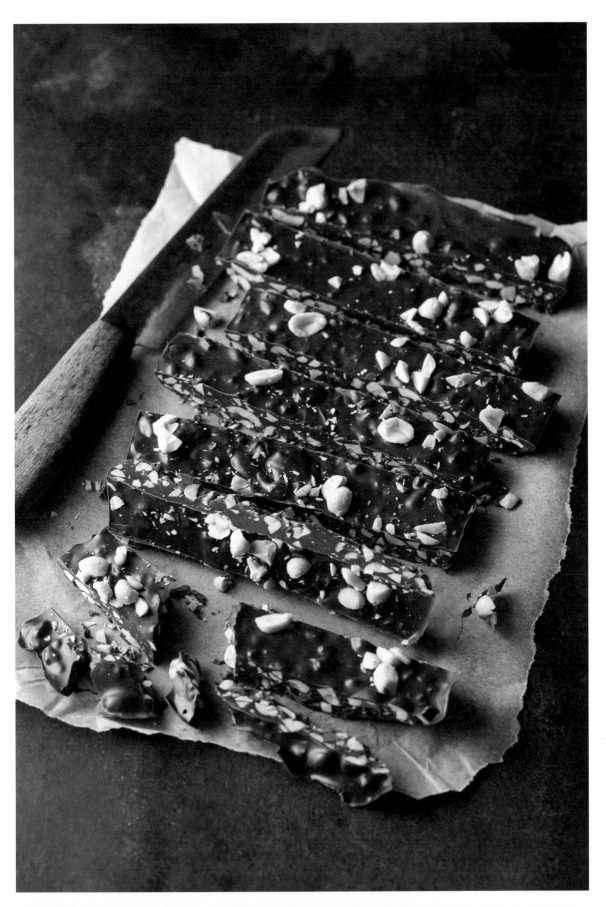

ALMOND AND COCONUT COOKIES

75 g (2½ oz) butter
150 g (1⅔ cups) desiccated coconut
50 g (½ cup) ground almonds
2 medium egg yolk
1 medium egg
birch sugar (xylitol, optional)

Makes 15 cookies
Preparation: approx. 20 minutes
Baking: approx. 10 minutes
Per cookie: approx. 115 kcal, 1 g protein,
12 g fat, 1 g carbohydrate

Preheat the oven to 400°F. Line a baking tray with greaseproof paper. Melt the butter in a small pan. Combine the desiccated coconut and ground almonds with the egg yolks and egg in a bowl. Add the melted, slightly cooled butter and work everything together by hand. Add some birch sugar, if desired.

Scoop teaspoons of the cookie mix and roll into balls between the palms of your hands. Place them on the baking tray and flatten by hand until 8 mm (⅜ in) thick. Slide the tray into the centre of the oven and bake for 10 minutes until the cookies are brown at the edges. Remove and leave to cool completely on the tray.

NUTTY COCONUT COOKIES

If you've just run out of almonds, or you have leftovers of some other nuts from another recipe, these cookies are the ideal way to use them up. Any kind of nut you happen to have in the cupboard or that needs using up can be used instead of the almonds, just grind the whole nuts in a food processor.

AVOCADO AND CHOCOLATE ICE CREAM

(V)

1 banana, roughly chopped
1 avocado, peeled, destoned and roughly chopped
50 g (scant ¼ cup) crème fraîche
2 tablespoons cocoa powder
½ teaspoon vanilla powder
1 tablespoon creamed coconut
1 tablespoon cold coffee
birch sugar (xylitol, optional)

Serves 2
Preparation: approx. 10 minutes
Freezing: approx. 40 minutes
Per portion: approx. 530 kcal, 8 g protein, 49 g fat, 14 g carbohydrate

Add the banana, avocado and crème fraîche to the bowl of a food processor with the blade fitted. Freeze in this container for 40–50 minutes.

Remove the food processor bowl from the freezer. Add the cocoa powder, vanilla powder, creamed coconut and cold coffee and process well. Add some birch sugar to taste, if using. Serve straight away in two little bowls.

NO ICE-CREAM MAKER REQUIRED

Normally ice cream is made by stirring it constantly in an ice-cream maker while it is being chilled. That isn't possible when making this ice cream. To make sure the ingredients don't get warm too quickly when you blend them, it really helps if the food processor bowl and blade have been frozen too. It's worth making a bit of extra room to do this in your freezer compartment. But be careful, ice cream can be addictive.

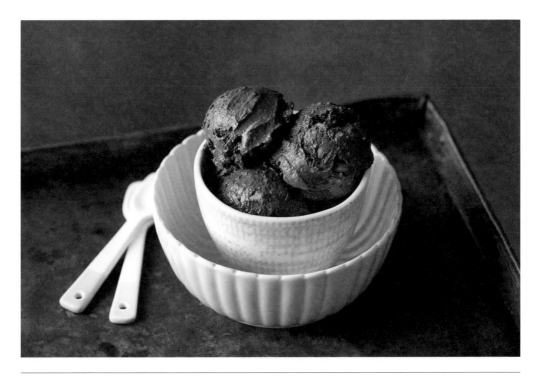

BULLETPROOF COFFEE

5 tablespoons ground coffee
8 teaspoons butter
3 tablespoons coconut oil

Serves 2
Preparation: approx. 10 minutes
Per serving: approx. 325 kcal, 7 g protein,
32 g fat, 1 g carbohydrate

Prepare two cups of coffee using 400 ml (1¾ cups) water and the ground coffee. Melt the butter and coconut oil in a pan over a medium heat and warm them slightly.

Add the coffee, butter and coconut oil to a blender and process until all the ingredients are combined and there is a nice layer of foam. Pour into two pre-warmed cups to serve.

FOR MORE INDULGENCE

You can jazz up this coffee with some vanilla powder, ground cinnamon or cardamom. If you have a sweet tooth, you can use a sweetener of your choice or just dissolve a little piece of dark chocolate (minimum 70 % cocoa content) in your coffee. If you like cream with your coffee, warm it up together with the butter and coconut oil.

BULLETPROOF HOT CHOCOLATE

(V)

200 g (generous ¾ cup) coconut milk
    (tinned)
5½ teaspoons soft butter
3 teaspoons coconut oil
4 tablespoons cocoa powder
¼ teaspoons vanilla powder
pinch of ground cinnamon

Serves 2
Preparation: approx. 10 minutes
Per serving: approx. 510 kcal, 12 g
protein, 49 g fat, 6 g carbohydrate

Add the coconut milk to a small pan with 200 ml (¾ cup) water
and bring to the boil. Stir in the butter, coconut oil, cocoa
powder, vanilla and cinnamon and remove the pan from the heat.

Pour the hot chocolate into a blender and process until all the
ingredients have combined and there is a nice layer of foam.
Pour into two pre-warmed cups to serve.

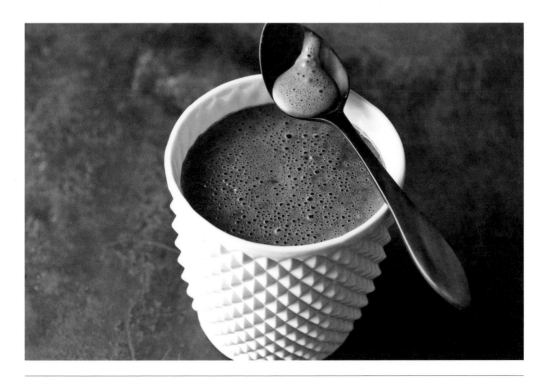

GENERAL INDEX

RECIPE INDEX

This Wind-Up Books edition published in 2019 by Elwin Street Productions Limited

Copyright © Elwin Street Productions Limited 2019

Conceived and produced by Elwin Street Limited
14 Clerkenwell Green
London EC1R 0DP
www.elwinstreet.com

ISBN 978-1-912827-09-1

Photography by Mona Binner, except p.22 (Shutterstock)
Translated from the original German edition (Gräfe und Unzer Verlag, 2017) by Alison Tunley

DISCLAIMER
The advice, recipes and meal plans in this book are intended as a personal guide to healthy living. However, this information is not intended to provide medical advice and should not replace the guidance of a qualified physician or other healthcare professional. Decisions about your health should be made by you and your healthcare provider based on the specific circumstances of your health, risk factors, family history and other considerations. See your healthcare provider before making major dietary changes or embarking on an exercise program, especially if you have existing health problems, medical conditions or chronic diseases. The author and publishers have made every effort to ensure that the information in this book is safe and accurate, but they cannot accept liability for any resulting injury or loss or damage to either property or person, whether direct or consequential and howsoever arising.

10 9 8 7 6 5 4 3 2 1

Printed in China